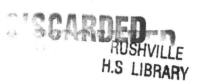

DECODING LIFE

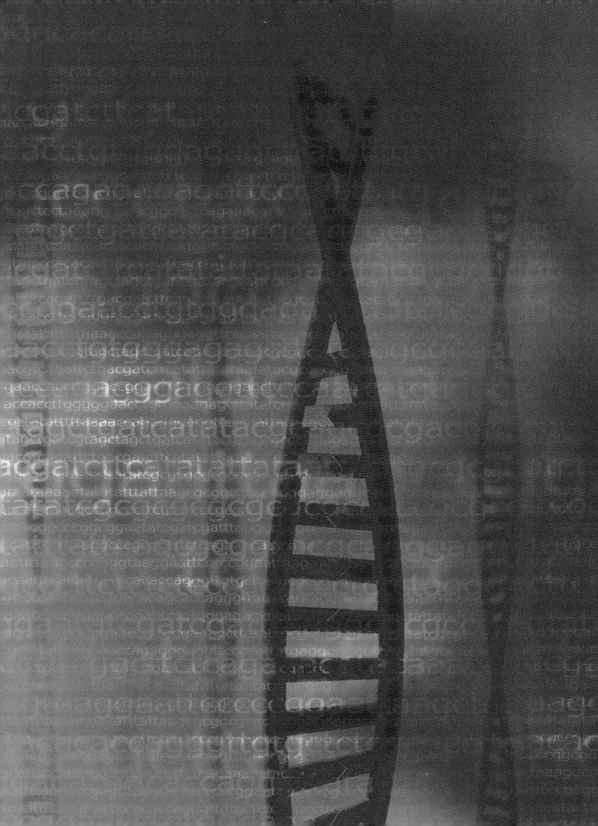

DECODING LIFE

UNRAVELING THE MYSTERIES OF THE GENOME

BY RON FRIDELL

LERNER PUBLICATIONS COMPANY
MINNEAPOLIS

The author would like to thank Dr. Rex Chisholm, director of the Center for Genetic Medicine at Northwestern University's Feinberg School of Medicine in Chicago, for his clear, concise, and plain-spoken views on various aspects of genetic research, and Karina L. Briley, a genetic counselor at Yale University's Cancer Genetic Counseling Center in New Haven, Connecticut, for reviewing early versions of the manuscript. The author also would like to thank Melissa Stewart and Carol Hinz for their expert work in shaping and refining this book.

Pages 2–3: an illustration of DNA (foreground), the molecule that contains genetic information and is passed from parent to child during reproduction. DNA is shaped like a double helix (spiraling ladder) and is housed in the nucleus of most cells. The letters A, C, T, and G (background) stand for the four nucleotide bases of DNA. See pages 14–17 for more information.

Lerner Publications Company
A Division of Lerner Publishing Group
241 First Avenue North
Minneapolis, Minnesota 55401 U.S.A.

Website address: www.lernerbooks.com

Library of Congress Cataloging-in-Publication Data

Fridell, Ron.
    Decoding life: unraveling the mysteries of the genome / written by Ron Fridell.
       p.   cm. — (Discovery!)
    Includes bibliographical references and index.
    ISBN: 0–8225–1196–7 (lib. bdg. : alk. paper)
    1. Genetics—Juvenile literature. I. Title.
  QH437.5.F7485 2005
  611'.018166—dc22   2004004710

Manufactured in the United States of America
1 2 3 4 5 6 – JR – 10 09 08 07 06 05

CONTENTS

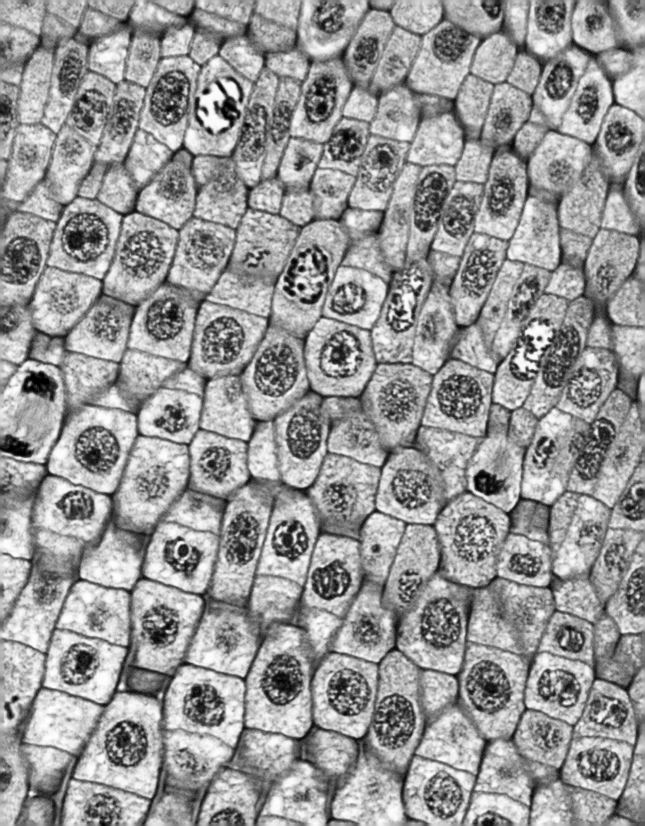

INTRODUCTION

Imagine this: you possess a guide to the most precious, most mysterious secrets of life.

Actually, you don't have to imagine. You really do have such a guide. It's a genetic manual that explains in detail how to build and operate a human being. But this guide to your genetic material, known as the human genome, isn't something you can hold in your hands or read with your eyes. It's incredibly tiny and is buried deep inside you. Nearly every one of the 100 trillion cells in your body holds a complete copy of this operating manual for a human being—you.

Each copy of your genome is alike, but your genome is also unique. No one else on Earth has a genome exactly like yours. In fact, every living thing—from viruses to dandelions to whales—has its own unique genome.

Over the last fifty years, scientists and researchers have learned how to decode and understand more and more of the human genome. A great deal of work remains to be done. As scientists continue to unravel the mysteries of the genome, they will gain vast new knowledge. Over the next few decades, this knowledge will put enormous new powers at our command.

Some experts predict that we will use these new powers wisely and well. We will use them to cure and prevent diseases, to lengthen human life, to make ourselves stronger and healthier, to feed hungry people, to save endangered species, and a great

A microscopic view of human skin cells, stained with dye to make their structures visible *(facing page)*. The dark center, or nucleus, of each cell holds a copy of this person's genome, a complete set of genetic material.

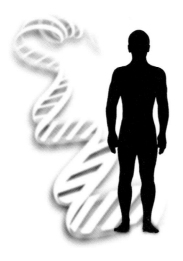
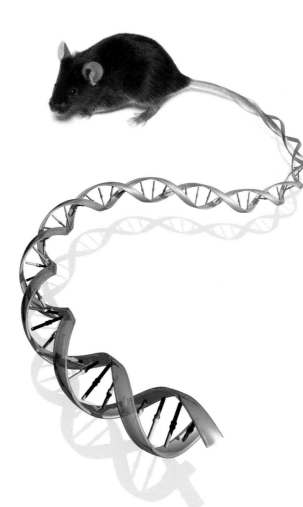

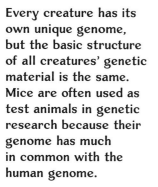

Every creature has its own unique genome, but the basic structure of all creatures' genetic material is the same. Mice are often used as test animals in genetic research because their genome has much in common with the human genome.

deal more. In their eyes, the genomic revolution will lead us toward a future filled with glorious promises.

Other experts see things very differently. They warn that our good intentions could lead to unintended consequences. As scientists experiment with the genomes of plants and animals, they will perform tens of thousands of complex operations on all sorts of living things. During these experiments, they will alter the most vital and delicate part of any organism, its genome. What if the experiments do not turn out as planned? What if scientists end up creating menacing new plants and animals that upset the balance of nature? What if their attempts to improve our own species lead to an elite superrace that discriminates against the rest of us? This book traces the genomic revolution and examines the promises and perils that it holds in store for each and every one of us.

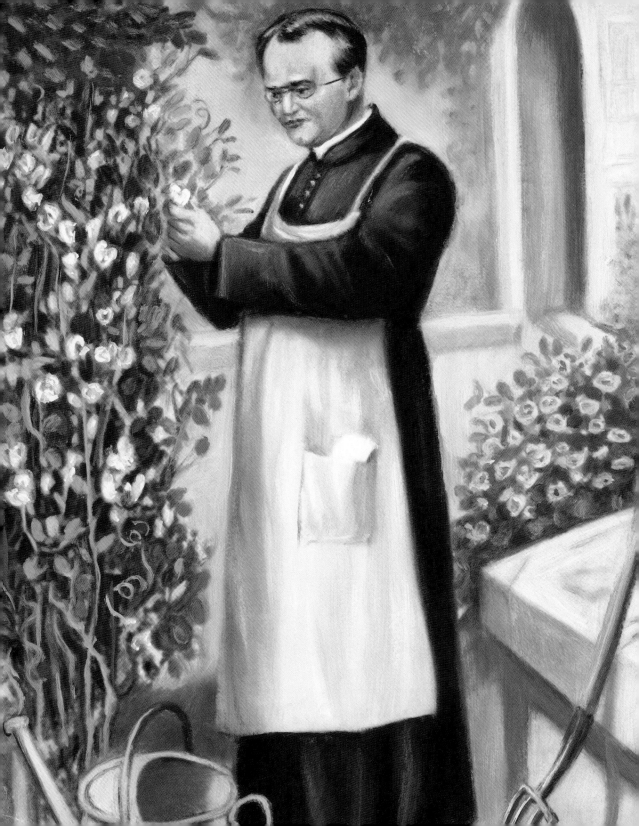

Chapter One

EXPLORING THE UNKNOWN

In a way, the scientists who discovered the genome were like the early explorers who set out on sailing ships for uncharted lands or the first astronauts in outer space. The genomic explorers were headed in a different direction, though. They were exploring the uncharted lands deep inside the human body.

Many scientists took part in these early explorations. Looking back, three names in particular stand out: Crick, Watson, and Franklin. Francis Crick was a British biophysicist, James Watson was an American biologist, and Rosalind Franklin was a British chemist. All three worked at university laboratories in England in the early 1950s. In 1953 Crick and Franklin were in their thirties, and Watson was just twenty-five years old.

Thanks to the work of earlier researchers, the three scientists knew the basics of genetics. In the 1800s, an Austrian monk named Gregor Mendel had begun experimenting with pea plants. He bred plants with different characteristics (such as different pea colors) to study how the plants passed along those characteristics from one generation to the next. In the early 1900s, other scientists noticed the importance of Mendel's work. They conducted additional experiments with other plants and with animals. They determined that the traits of plants and animals are passed along by genes. Genes are part of larger units called chromosomes that are found in the nucleus of most plant and animal cells.

Gregor Mendel *(facing page)* **conducted his pea-plant experiments at the Austrian monastery where he lived in the mid-1800s.**

Although chromosomes are small, the scientists were able to see them under the microscope. Their microscopes were not powerful enough to show the genes. The scientists learned that humans have twenty-three pairs of chromosomes. These chromosomes contain all of our genetic material—our genome.

Scientists determined that a copy of the human genome is found in nearly every cell of the body. Chemical analysis revealed that the genome is recorded in a substance called deoxyribonucleic acid (DNA). DNA holds the secrets to how the body manufactures cells, how the body operates, and how it eventually breaks down and dies.

These discoveries set the stage for the work of Crick, Watson, and Franklin. To learn more, these scientists needed to figure out DNA's structure.

Crick and Watson worked as a team. They didn't have a way to look at DNA molecules directly, but they could make deductions, or educated guesses, based on their research. Crick and Watson used their deductions to build a cardboard model of how they thought the DNA molecule might be shaped. But the model was rough. They needed more information to fill in the gaps.

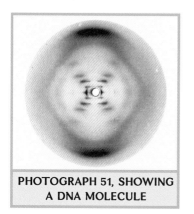

PHOTOGRAPH 51, SHOWING A DNA MOLECULE

Meanwhile, Rosalind Franklin was working in another laboratory, using a different strategy. She was skilled at photographing microorganisms—objects so small that they could be seen only with a microscope. Her photography technique was called X-ray crystallography. With this technique, Franklin produced Photograph 51, an X-ray image of a molecule of DNA.

2) THE CELL: Cells are the building blocks of the human body. While different cells have many different functions, they all contain the same basic components.

3) THE NUCLEUS: In the center of most cells lies the nucleus. It is the control center, telling every other part of the cell what to do.

1) THE BODY: The human body contains about 100 trillion cells. To isolate DNA, scientists must look deep inside cells.

4) THE CHROMOSOME: Within the nucleus of a human cell are twenty-three chromosomes. Together, these chromosomes hold all of a person's genetic information. Chromosomes are made up of very tightly coiled deoxyribonucleic acid (DNA).

5) DNA: DNA forms an interconnected, spiral shape known as a double helix. DNA contains the human genome—all of the information required to make and operate a human being. Sections of DNA that code for (determine) genetic traits passed from parent to child are known as genes.

ZOOM IN ON DNA

When Crick and Watson saw Photograph 51, it showed them exactly what they'd been missing. "The instant I saw the picture," Watson said, "my mouth fell open and my heart began to race." The picture gave them the vital information they needed to complete their DNA model.

UNDERSTANDING DNA

On February 28, 1953, Crick and Watson burst into the Eagle Pub, a tavern in Cambridge, England, and boldly announced to one and all that they had "found the secret of life." Two months later, they published the first detailed description of the DNA molecule in the British science magazine *Nature*. Their article was titled, "Molecular Structure of Nucleic Acids." While their announcement in the pub had been brash and dramatic, their article was modest and formal. They wrote that they believed their discovery would be "of considerable biological interest."

Their discovery, of course, meant far more than that. Thanks to them, the world knows the basic structure of DNA. It looks like a spiraling ladder, a shape sometimes called a double helix. This double helix is made of building blocks called nucleotides.

Each nucleotide has three parts—a phosphate group, a sugar, and a base. The phosphate group of one nucleotide bonds to the sugar of another to form the sides of the ladder. The rungs, or steps, are formed when the bases of neighboring nucleotides bond together.

Based on the discoveries of other scientists, Crick and Watson knew that DNA contained four nitrogenous bases, represented by the letters A, T, C, and G. These bases are the molecules adenine (A), thymine (T), cytosine (C), and guanine (G).

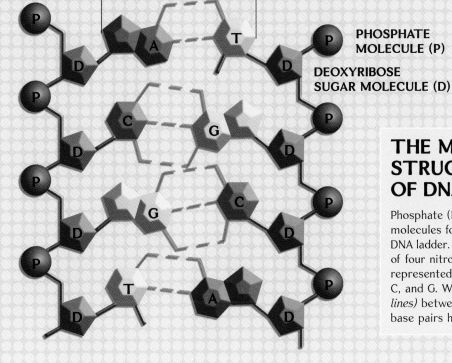

NITROGENOUS BASES (A, T, C, AND G)

PHOSPHATE MOLECULE (P)

DEOXYRIBOSE SUGAR MOLECULE (D)

THE MOLECULAR STRUCTURE OF DNA

Phosphate (P) and sugar (D) molecules form the sides of the DNA ladder. The rungs are made of four nitrogenous bases, represented by the letters A, T, C, and G. Weak bonds *(dotted lines)* between the A–T and C–G base pairs hold DNA together.

Each of these bases has a partner, another base that it always pairs with to form a rung on the ladder. Base A always bonds with base T, and C always joins with G. These A-T and C-G partners are known as base pairs.

This DNA ladder is the human genome. It tells the body what to do by programming the body's cells to produce proteins, the basic components of life. Proteins are the building blocks that make up our cells, organs, and tissues.

Once scientists knew this much about the genome, their next task was clear. They needed to decode the genome to find out how DNA directs cells to make proteins. There was a problem, though—a huge one. No one—not even Crick, Watson, or Franklin—knew how to determine the order of the bases making up the genome, let alone how to decipher what the order meant.

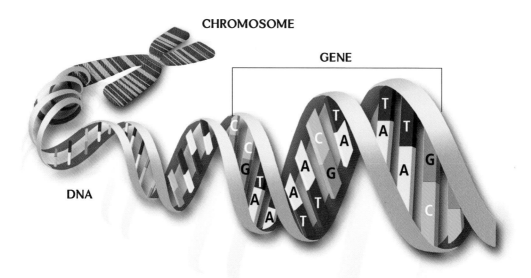

CHROMOSOME

GENE

DNA

This illustration shows a sequence of working base pairs, or a gene. Genes instruct the body to make proteins that help cells form, grow, and work. The human genome contains about 3 billion base pairs but not all form genes.

GENES AND PROTEINS

As scientists continued to study DNA, they realized that certain groups of base pairs work together. These working groups, or sequences, of base pairs are called genes. The base pairs that make up each gene spell out the recipe for making one or more proteins. Since these protein recipes are the keys to understanding how the body grows and works, scientists worked on decoding the genes. The process of decoding genes is known as sequencing. It amounts to listing the sequence, or order, of base pairs in a gene, from start to finish.

At first glance, the job of sequencing the human genome doesn't sound all that difficult. After all, when the genome is fully unraveled, it's just 6 feet (2 meters) long and less than .004

of an inch (.1 millimeter) wide. That doesn't seem like much territory to cover. But when you look at the human genome as scientists do—on a microscopic level—you see that it's truly vast. The genome contains tens of thousands of genes, and the instructions for building a single protein could be one, 1,000, 100,000, or even 1 million base pairs long.

THE HUMAN GENOME PROJECT

Even though the job looked overwhelming, scientists were determined to sequence the entire human genome. Their goal began to seem more realistic in the mid-1980s, when rapid advances in computer and medical technology gave them the tools they needed. In October 1990, the U.S. Department of Energy (DOE) and the National Institutes of Health (NIH) officially launched the Human Genome Project (HGP)—an international effort to sequence the entire human genome by the year 2005. The U.S. government gave DOE and NIH billions of dollars to fund research projects that would help them reach their goal.

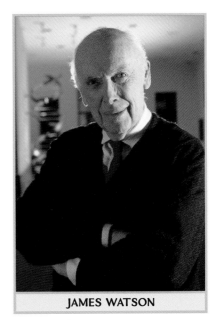

JAMES WATSON

DNA pioneer James Watson headed the HGP. He assembled and supervised teams of scientists in the United States, the United Kingdom, France, Germany, and Japan. As the project got under way, the scientists first focused their attention on creating a basic "map" of the genome. They identified major reference points along the chromosomes. Later, they would go back and fill in the thousands of base pairs between the reference points.

In 1992 Watson retired and Francis Collins took over as head of the HGP. Collins was a geneticist known for his fast, accurate work in locating genes. The project continued to move along according to plan until 1998. Then a new team entered the picture, and the project turned into a race. This new team was Celera, a biotechnology company in Rockville, Maryland. Celera had been founded by Craig Venter, an unlikely sort of person to head a biotech company. Venter nearly flunked out of high school, spent his time surfing instead of going to college, and then served in the Vietnam War. After the war ended in the mid-1970s, he enrolled in college and earned his Ph.D.

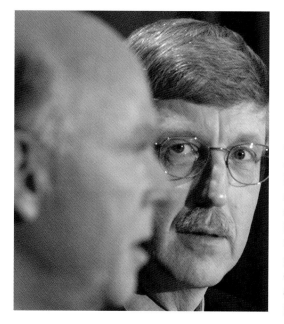

Craig Venter of Celera *(left)* **and Francis Collins of the HGP** *(right)* **speak to reporters about their progress in decoding the human genome. Even though Venter and Collins ran competing projects, the two men often appeared together at scientific meetings and press conferences.**

He specialized in biomedical research and eventually became a scientist-entrepreneur. Venter boldly announced that Celera, not the HGP, would produce the first complete draft of the human genome.

Venter's reasons for sequencing the genome were different from the HGP's. The HGP was a nonprofit venture funded by the federal government. It would make no money from its discoveries. HGP scientists worked strictly for the good of humanity. The HGP posted its sequence on the Internet, granting free access to scientists—and anyone else who wanted to see it—around the world.

Celera, however, was in the race for another motive—profit. According to Venter, the company would create a database of genes and then sell access to the database to drug companies and researchers. Many investors liked what they heard about Celera, and they poured millions of dollars into the new company. This money was exactly what Venter needed to get his ambitious project up and running. The race was on.

The two teams worked in different ways. HGP scientists proceeded slowly and methodically, moving through the long DNA ladder piece by piece. First, they broke a small section into fragments. Then they used high-tech machines known as sequencers to "read" the series of base pairs in each fragment. Finally, they carefully returned each sequenced section to its original location on the DNA ladder. The deliberate HGP process ensured that their data were extremely accurate.

The HGP had an eight-year head start, so Celera scientists had to work faster to catch up. But Venter had a plan. His team would use a method called whole-genome shotgun sequencing. Celera scientists broke the genome into larger fragments and used more sequencer machines than the HGP scientists.

HOW TO SEQUENCE A GENOME

Both the HGP labs and Celera used the same five steps to sequence the human genome: chopping, cloning, tagging, re-sorting, and reading.

1. DNA is chopped into fragments.

2. Each fragment is soaked in a special solution of bacteria that causes the DNA to clone, or copy, itself millions of times. This process gives scientists plenty of cloned copies to work with.

3. The cloned fragments are fed into chemical solutions for tagging. The nucleotides at the ends of each fragment get their own fluorescent tags. The fluorescent tags make each base-pair letter—A, T, C, G— turn a different color when viewed under special lighting.

4. Computers sort the tagged fragments and return them to their proper location on the DNA ladder.

5. A laser in a DNA sequencer machine reads each tag and shows scientists the order of base-pair letters that make up the fragment.

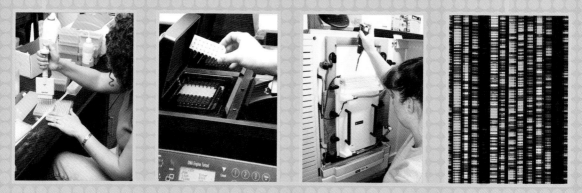

The DNA sequencing process (from left to right): DNA fragments are fed into a bacterial solution (image 1); chemically treated DNA fragments are placed in a thermal cycler for fluorescent tagging (image 2); a DNA sequencer reads the tagged DNA (image 3); and a computer image of the sequenced base pairs (image 4).

In addition, Celera created a computer program that would reassemble the entire genome back into the correct order at the end of the sequencing process.

When Collins and his HGP scientists saw how much their rival had picked up the pace, they began using Celera's sequencing techniques. But the HGP scientists also realized they needed to speed up their work without sacrificing accuracy. They set a goal of creating a rough draft of the entire genome as quickly as possible. Then they could double-check their work to create a highly accurate final draft. If the HGP and Celera had been racehorses, their noses would have hit the finish line at exactly the same moment. In June 2000, the race to produce a rough draft of the human genome ended in a tie—five years ahead of the original HGP schedule.

THE FINAL DRAFT

After completing the rough draft, HGP scientists began phase two of their plan: filling in gaps and fixing errors in the rough draft. Celera, meanwhile, decided to focus its attention elsewhere. Even so, the HGP scientists kept up their fast pace. Sixteen different research institutions located all over the world cooperated to get the job done.

The HGP scientists finished well ahead of the 2005 deadline. The final draft was published in April 2003—just in time for the fiftieth anniversary of Crick and Watson's landmark article on the structure of DNA. The human genome had been sequenced at a cost of $3 billion—fifty cents for every human being on Earth.

The final draft was approximately three billion nucleotide bases long. If the letters used to represent the base pairs were written out on paper, they would fill several hundred phone directories. To type them all, a person would have to work eight hours a day for *fifty years,* typing at a speed of sixty words per minute. Because the human genome is so huge, scientists will need to study it for many years to understand it completely. But even a quick look at the final draft revealed important and surprising information.

The biggest surprise was the number of genes—the DNA sequences that code for particular proteins. When the Human Genome Project began, scientists expected to find between 80,000 and 140,000 genes. Instead, the final draft revealed only about 30,000. The draft also showed that no two genes are the same size. They vary from a few hundred bases to a few million, with an average length of about three thousand base pairs.

Another surprise was the amount of space genes occupy. Scientists knew genes take up only a small part of the genome, but it turns out they occupy even less space than expected. According to the final draft, genes take up less than 2 percent of the genome.

The other 98 percent of the genome is known as "junk DNA." For many years, scientists thought this "junk" was the remains of the body's failed attempts to make genes. Experts compared the genome to a desert landscape—vast, barren stretches of "junk DNA" with genes scattered here and there like lush oases.

As researchers looked more closely, they saw that the "junk" was not so useless after all. True, it doesn't code for proteins, but some of it appears to be useful in other ways. For example, some "junk" sequences, known as promoters, turn genes on and off to control the amount of proteins a cell manufactures.

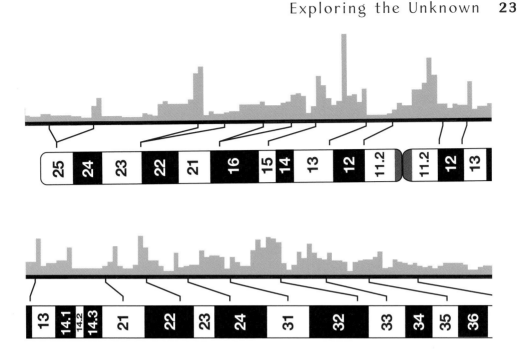

The image above is a map depicting some of the genes on chromosome 2. The orange graphs show the concentration of genes along the chromosome, with the higher bars indicating more genes. The numbers on the chromosome are location markers, much like milepost markers along a highway.

Scientists believe they will discover other important uses for this "junk" in years to come.

Scientists sometimes compare the final draft of the genome to a map. This map gives researchers the tool they have craved since Crick and Watson first published their description of DNA. Before the genome map, genetic researchers had only scattered bits and pieces of information to work with. Now they have a framework. Every new discovery they make will fit into this framework somewhere, and each new discovery will make the human genome a little bit less of a mystery.

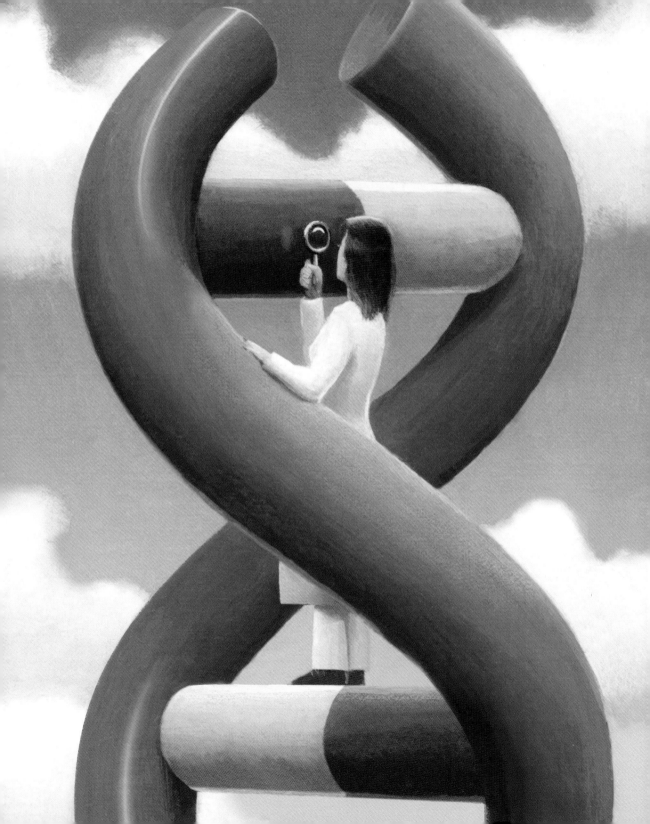

Chapter Two

SEARCHING FOR DAMAGED GENES

Many serious diseases are gene-based. They are caused partly or wholly by damaged genes. With a complete map of the human genome, scientists can search for these faulty genes. "We're trying to find the mechanisms underlying illness," said Eric Lander, a researcher at Whitehead Institute in Cambridge, Massachusetts. "We don't know what causes asthma, diabetes, hypertension, heart disease. Now we stand a real chance of knowing how to address all the major diseases."

The key to finding damaged genes is finding mutations. *Mutant* is a familiar word to comic book and science fiction fans. Spider-Man, the Hulk, and the X-Men are all mutants— humans transformed by changes to their genomes. The rampaging giant ants and spiders in science fiction movies are mutants too, transformed by doses of radiation or toxic chemicals into monstrous, evil creatures.

In real life, mutant genes have nothing to do with superpowers, but they do have one thing in common with science fiction mutants. They have been transformed by mutations. A mutation is a change in a gene's sequence of base-pair letters, a kind of spelling mistake. Genes can mutate for all sorts of reasons, including ultraviolet radiation from the sun, cosmic rays from outer space,

Researchers are closely examining the human genome, as pictured on the facing page, hoping to find the causes of genetic diseases. Changes, or mutations, in DNA sequence can lead to disease.

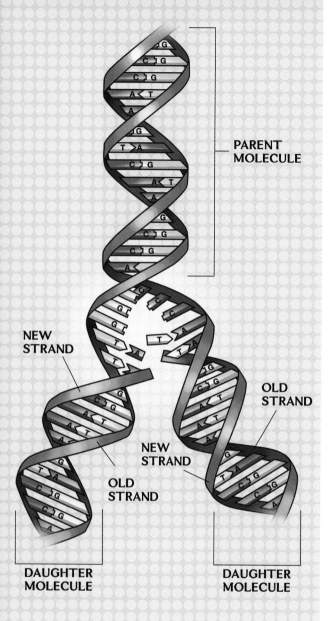

PARENT
MOLECULE

NEW
STRAND

OLD
STRAND

NEW
STRAND

OLD
STRAND

DAUGHTER
MOLECULE

DAUGHTER
MOLECULE

DNA REPLICATION

When DNA replicates, or copies itself, the original strands of DNA split apart to generate new complementary strands. The original DNA is known as the parent molecule, and the two new sets of DNA—each containing one old strand and one new strand—are called daughter molecules.

exhaust fumes from diesel engines, and smoke from cigarettes. Mutations can also be random and accidental, with no clearly apparent cause.

Most mutations occur during replication, when a cell divides in two as part of natural human growth. The entire DNA ladder "unzips" down the middle, and each base-pair rung splits in half. This leaves two separate and incomplete halves. The DNA then generates a new, complementary half for each incomplete half. That way, the body's new cells have DNA that matches the rest of the DNA in the body.

Almost always, the result is two complete, identical DNA ladders. Each new DNA molecule is an exact replica of the original. But sometimes things go wrong. Nucleotide bases get reversed or deleted or duplicated, and mutations occur.

Instantly, most mutations are corrected by a special class

of enzymes called repair enzymes. Enzymes are a type of protein. But repair enzymes don't catch every mistake. Some mutations survive. A DNA molecule doesn't know that surviving mutations are mistakes, so the next time it copies itself, the mutations get copied too. These surviving mutations become a permanent part of a person's genome, and over time, they build up. Scientists estimate that the average person accumulates about one hundred new mutations during a lifetime. Most of these mutations are harmless, and some are actually helpful. But a few mutations can be harmful—even fatal.

Harmful mutations trigger disease. Remember that each gene spells out a code for a protein recipe, and mutations may change that code. When they do, the mutated gene may produce damaged proteins or stop producing proteins entirely. If a protein isn't made or can't do its job, a disease may develop.

DECODING DISEASES

Armed with the map of the genome, scientists such as Eric Lander search for disease-causing mutations. They know that the mutations lie somewhere within the genomes of patients who have the same disease. The scientists take DNA samples from several people afflicted with a disease and carefully compare their genomes, searching for mutations that these patients share. These shared mutations, located in the same gene in each patient's genome, are highly likely to play a key role in causing the disease. This search for mutant genes is known as genotyping. Looking for shared mutations in different genomes takes a great deal of time and patience, but uncovering them is the first step in finding a cure for the disease they trigger.

Scientists started using genotyping even before the human genome was completely sequenced. As early as the 1980s, researchers discovered mutations responsible for single-gene disorders, diseases in which mutations on a single gene do all the damage.

Huntington's disease is an example of a single-gene disorder. In 1993 scientists pinpointed the location of the gene with the Huntington's mutation on chromosome 4.

Huntington's is a disease of the central nervous system: the brain, spinal cord, and spinal nerves. Most patients notice their first symptoms, losing their balance more than normal or slurring their speech, at about the age of forty. As time passes, they begin to lose control of all their muscles. Patients usually die before the age of fifty-five. Huntington's disease remains an incurable condition, but locating the single-gene mutation that causes it was the first step in someday finding a cure.

The mutation that causes Huntington's disease is a repetition of the bases CAG in a gene called *HD*. If these bases are repeated only a few times, no harm is done. But when they're repeated more than about thirty-eight times, the person carrying the mutated gene is almost certain to get the disease. The more CAG repeats a person has, the younger that person will likely be when he or she begins experiencing the first Huntington's symptoms.

In some ways, the scientists studying Huntington's disease are fortunate because they can focus all their attention on one particular gene. A genome with the mutation that causes Huntington's disease is like a car engine with a single problem. Let's say that problem is a faulty fuel pump. If you can fix the fuel pump, the engine will run fine. Similarly, if scientists can find a way to repair the gene with the Huntington's mutation, the disease will be cured.

← *HD* GENE

16

15.3
15.2
15.1
14

12

12

13.1
13.2
13.3

21.1
21.2
21.3

22

23

24

24

26

27

28

31.1
31.1
31.3

32

33

34

35

CHROMOSOME 4

The gene with the mutation that causes Huntington's disease (HD)—which affects the brain and central nervous system— is located at the very tip of chromosome 4. The light and dark bands on the chromosome map at left correspond to bands that appear when human chromosome 4 is stained with dye. The bands appear because the structure of the chromosome is not uniform. The denser parts have more tightly packed base pairs. These parts take up more dye and turn a darker color.

Most genetic diseases are much more complicated. They involve several mutations on several different genes. A genome with a multigene disorder is like a car engine that has a dozen different things wrong with it. Christopher Stodgell, a scientist at the University of Rochester in Rochester, New York, compares multigene diseases to an orchestra whose members are out of sync. When the musicians in the orchestra play the wrong notes at the wrong times, the music sounds awful. Something similar happens when a person has a multigene disease. When several mutant genes stop making the proper proteins to do the right jobs at the right times, the person's body stops working properly.

The mutations that cause multigene diseases tend to be scattered all over the genome, so it's hard to find them all. But before scientists can hope to cure a multigene disease, they must locate each of the mutant genes involved.

One common multigene disease is asthma, a condition that affects breathing. So far, scientists have identified more than fifteen different mutant genes that may contribute to asthma. One of them, *ADAM33*, is located on chromosome 20. One research study found that 40 percent of asthma sufferers have mutant versions of the *ADAM33* gene. While asthma attacks can be triggered by air pollution, tobacco smoke, and other outside irritants, *ADAM33* and other mutant genes seem to play a significant role by increasing sensitivity to these irritants. Researchers continue their search for other genes that contribute to asthma. Finding the genes will help them develop new treatments.

THE QUEST TO CURE CANCER

Asthma is seldom fatal, but some multigene disorders are. One of these is cancer, a group of diseases that occur when people's cells start growing out of control. Cancer kills about half a million Americans every year, so it's high on the list of genetic diseases that scientists want to cure.

Before researchers can cure cancer, they must locate the damaged genes responsible for the disease. To do this, scientists use genotyping. They compare the genomes of patients with the same kind of cancer and search for shared mutations.

Researchers have discovered that most cancer-related mutations cause certain genes to get stuck in the "on" position. What does this mean? Healthy genes work for a while, then

Scientists have located a gene on chromosome 17 that leads to some forms of breast cancer *(right center)*. More research may produce a cure or lifesaving treatments for this life–threatening disease.

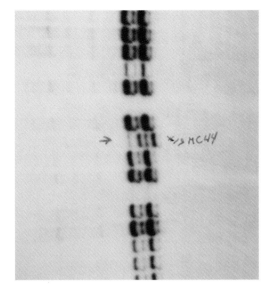

they rest, and then they work some more. But cancer-causing mutations program genes to keep on working all the time, day and night. Because the mutant genes are stuck in the "on" position, they never stop making proteins.

A gene that can mutate to trigger cancer is called an oncogene. When an oncogene is healthy, it does a vital job. It makes sure the body generates new tissue to heal wounds and keep growing. But when oncogenes mutate, they instruct cells to produce more new tissue than the body needs. Over time, the extra tissue piles up and forms a cancerous growth known as a tumor.

But damaged oncogenes are only half of the cancer problem. Damaged tumor suppressor genes are the other half. Tumor suppressor genes stop runaway tissue growth. The gene *TP53* is a tumor suppressor gene nicknamed the guardian angel of the genome. The moment that *TP53* detects out-of-control oncogenes, it tells cells to produce p53, a protein that destroys cancer cells. In more that half of all cancer patients, *TP53* has mutated in a way that stops protein production. When *TP53* gets stuck in the "off" position, it can't do its job, and cancer continues to spread.

Cancer cannot be cured until scientists learn how to shut off oncogenes stuck in the "on" position and switch on tumor suppressing genes stuck in the "off" position. This will take many years of closely studying the genome.

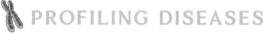 PROFILING DISEASES

Think of a wanted poster for a criminal. It shows the person's picture and lists vital statistics such as age, height, and eye color. It also lists the crimes for which the criminal is wanted.

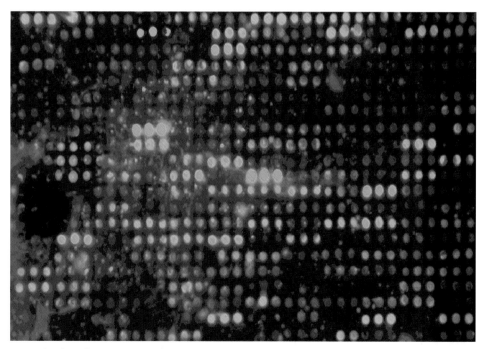

The bright spots on this DNA chip help identify the DNA donor's active genes. Scientists and doctors use DNA chips to check for disease-causing genes.

Try to imagine a wanted poster for a disease. What would it look like? Sometimes the scientists studying a particular disease create a profile, a kind of wanted poster for that condition. It tells what causes the disease and shows how the disease does its damage. Once scientists have profiled a disease, they can work on finding a cure.

A multigene disease is hard to profile because the mutant genes involved are scattered through the genome. To trigger the disease, these genes must all fail to do their jobs at the same time. To profile a multigene disease, scientists need a way to see all the mutant genes in operation at once. To get this view, they use a tool called a DNA microarray, a piece of glass the size of a dime infused with genetic material. It is also known as a DNA chip. A DNA chip is made of tens of thousands of DNA sequences stuck to the glass surface. An unknown DNA sequence from a patient will bind to the spot on the chip that has that same sequence, enabling researchers to identify it. Using DNA chips, researchers can identify thousands of DNA sequences that are active in a person's genome at a given moment.

Once scientists identify which of a patient's genes are switched on, they ask a series of questions. What instructions do the active genes carry? Are the genes working properly? If not, what part do the genes play in causing disease? Scientists use the answers to these questions to build a disease profile.

To build a complete profile, scientists must see all the genes in a person's genome at once. Early gene chips could hold only some of a person's genes. But during 2003 and 2004, several biotech companies made breakthroughs. They produced chips that could hold all of the 30,000 or so genes in a person's genome. Finally, researchers could see a complete genomic profile to help them find ways to repair mutant genes and cure the diseases they trigger.

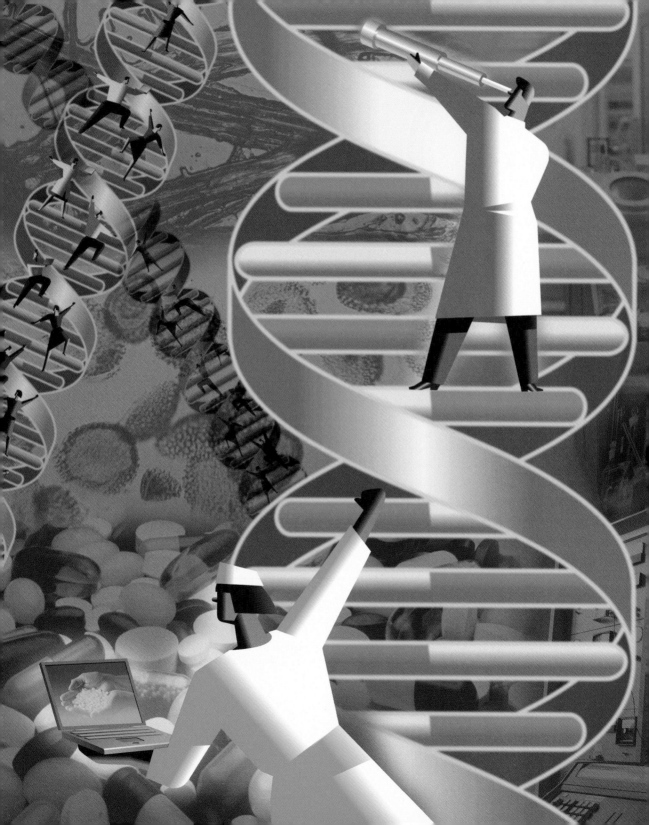

Chapter Three

REPAIRING DAMAGED GENES

Since the beginning of medicine, patients with genetic diseases have been treated according to their symptoms. Symptoms are noticeable changes in the working of the body that signal a disease or illness. Sneezing, a sore throat, coughing, and headaches are symptoms of the common cold—a viral infection. When you have a cold, you take medicines to relieve the symptoms until the cold goes away.

Similarly, patients with genetic diseases receive drugs and other forms of therapy to relieve the symptoms they suffer. For instance, cancer patients may receive radiation treatments to reduce pain and kill cancerous growths. Sometimes these treatments are successful in checking the damage. They may even cure the patient.

But even when a patient is cured, the disease itself isn't. Other people will continue to get the same disease. Scientists want to change all that. They hope to one day eliminate genetic diseases entirely. To achieve this amazing goal, researchers will rely on gene therapy, a radical new medical technique that aims to correct the errors in mutated genes.

In recent years, scientists have begun experimenting with gene therapy to repair the damaged genes of sick patients. One day, gene therapy may also be used to prevent genetic diseases

This image *(facing page)* is an artist's depiction of our fast-growing knowledge about the human genome and how that knowledge is helping doctors develop ways to genetically treat and repair damaged genes.

from ever developing. For this to happen, scientists would have to be able to thoroughly analyze a person's genome for disease-causing mutations. Then, in theory, they could repair the damaged genes before the person ever got sick. In other words, they would delete the disease from the person's genome forever. Of all the advances the Human Genome Project makes possible, gene therapy offers the most promising benefits for humankind.

The basic theory behind gene therapy is simple. Turning that theory into practice is much more challenging. The very first gene therapy techniques scientists have developed are still in the early experimental stages. They are conducted almost exclusively with test animals in laboratories. Very little work has been done with human subjects because the results are too risky, too unpredictable. The technology needed to make gene therapy a reality will take many years to develop. Still, many experts believe that eventually gene therapy will revolutionize the practice of medicine.

HOW GENE THERAPY WORKS

Most gene therapy researchers work with somatic cells. Somatic cells are all the cells in the body except egg cells and sperm cells. How does somatic gene therapy work? Basically, it's a matter of replacing damaged genes with healthy genes. "If you have a broken gene, doctors can give you a good copy of that gene to replace the broken one, and thereby cure the disease," explains geneticist Rex Chisholm, director of the Center for Genetic Medicine at Northwestern University's Feinberg School of Medicine in Chicago, Illinois.

The procedure sounds simple enough, but there's a catch. How do doctors deliver the replacement gene to the patient's cells? "This presents a big technical problem," Chisholm says. "If every cell in your body has that broken gene, how do you get that copy of the gene into every cell in your body?"

To find out, let's use a gene we're familiar with: the Huntington's gene on chromosome 4. The Huntington's gene codes for a protein manufactured in the brain. Patients with the mutated Huntington's gene make too much of this protein. How can scientists replace this damaged gene in every one of a patient's 100 billion or so brain cells?

The secret is designing a device that can deliver the new gene to its proper destination. Researchers are experimenting with several delivery devices. One that looks especially promising is called a vector. It's something like a tiny cargo ship. It transports a healthy gene to the genome and then unloads it. Scientists cannot yet control where in the genome the vector places the new gene, but it's something they hope to be able to figure out in the coming years. This step is extremely important because if a gene is inserted at the wrong point in the genome, it risks causing a new disease in the patient.

Many vectors are made from viruses. Normally, we think of a virus as something bad. After all, the tiny particles called viruses infect our bodies and cause diseases, such as the common cold, the flu, the measles, and acquired immunodeficiency syndrome (AIDS). But viruses are also skilled at invading the tiniest parts of the human body—including the genome. And that makes viral vectors good delivery devices.

Since gene therapy is in its early stages, nearly all the testing with viral vectors is done on animals. Before scientists insert the viruses into an animal's body, they alter them so they cannot cause diseases. But this harmless virus still has the ability to deliver its genetic cargo to repair damaged genes.

VIRUSES

A virus is a small piece of genetic material surrounded by a protective protein coat. A virus needs the help of a host cell to reproduce. When a virus enters the human body, it seeks out a cell to infect. The virus attaches itself to the outside wall of the host cell and inserts its genetic material into the cell. The new genetic material instructs the cell to stop its normal behavior and to start making copies of the virus. Eventually the cell bursts open and the new viruses move through the body, infecting more cells.

To use viral vectors (viruses carrying genetic material) in gene therapy, scientists must change two key parts of a virus's genome. First, they remove the part that makes people sick. Second, they remove the part that tells cells to make new copies of the virus. Then the scientists add the DNA sequence that they would like to insert into the genome of the patient undergoing gene therapy. As a result, the viral vector works only to get inside cells and insert the DNA that the patient's body needs.

A HUMAN SUCCESS STORY

Even though gene therapy is still risky and is in trial stages only, a few human patients have voluntarily undergone the procedure. These patients had life-threatening diseases that could not be treated with conventional medical techniques. Gene therapy was their only hope.

In September 1990, a four-year-old girl named Ashanthi "Ashi" DeSilva became the first person to successfully undergo gene therapy. Ashi was suffering from a form of a disease called severe combined immunodeficiency (SCID). Through genotyping, scientists discovered that her type of SCID is a single-gene disease triggered by a mutation in a gene known as *ADA*, on chromosome 20.

SCID is an extremely rare disease of the human immune system. Normally, the immune system protects the body against infections by fighting bacteria, viruses, and other invaders. Its most important weapons are white blood cells. When invaders enter the body, white blood cells usually attack and destroy them. But when the *ADA* gene is damaged, the body does not produce enough of a certain enzyme needed for the proper growth and function of white blood cells. As a result, people with SCID are in constant danger of dying from infections that a healthy immune system could fight off. Without treatment or isolation from germs, the life expectancy for a SCID patient is generally less than one year.

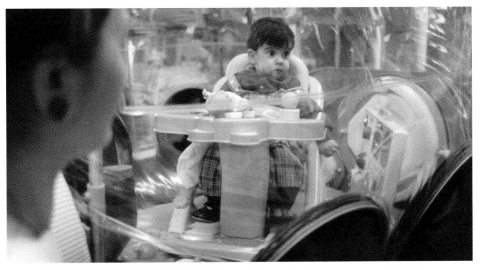

An infant suffering from SCID sits within a sterile room, or bubble. The infant's body cannot fight off infection, so she must be constantly protected from germs. In scientific trials, gene therapy has improved the health of SCID patients.

During Ashi's gene therapy, doctors extracted white blood cells from her body so they could treat them directly. Then they infected each cell with a viral vector containing the healthy *ADA* gene. Finally, they injected the genetically corrected white blood cells back into Ashi's bloodstream.

Shortly after the procedure, doctors saw the results they had hoped for. Ashi's immune system tripled its production of healthy white blood cells. The viral vectors had done their job. They had delivered healthy *ADA* genes to their proper place in Ashi's genome.

THE IMMUNE SYSTEM

The immune system protects the body against infection and disease. It fights antigens, or foreign substances, such as bacteria, viruses, and parasites. Immune cells known as white blood cells circulate throughout the body looking for antigens. When an antigen enters the body, the white blood cells identify it as an invader, surround the antigen, and destroy it. After fighting an antigen, white blood cells produce antibodies. Antibodies are proteins designed to fight a specific antigen that has previously invaded the body. If the antigen returns, the body recognizes it. The antibodies allow the body to respond more quickly to the antigen, preventing a person from becoming sick. If a person has a reduced number of white blood cells, caused by diseases such as SCID or AIDS, the body cannot fight infection very well, and the person will become sick more often. In some cases, the immune system overreacts to particular antigens, causing an allergic reaction. For some people, this reaction can be so severe that it leads to death.

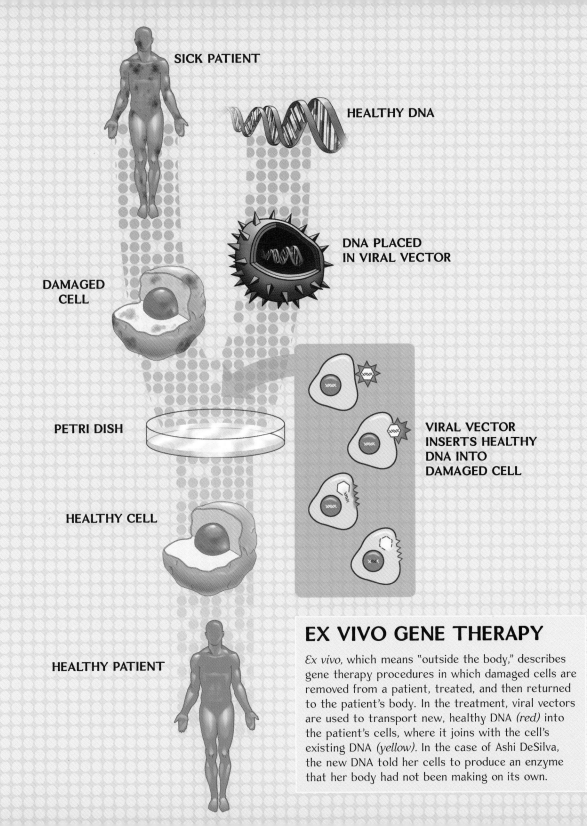

SICK PATIENT

HEALTHY DNA

DNA PLACED
IN VIRAL VECTOR

DAMAGED
CELL

PETRI DISH

VIRAL VECTOR
INSERTS HEALTHY
DNA INTO
DAMAGED CELL

HEALTHY CELL

HEALTHY PATIENT

EX VIVO GENE THERAPY

Ex vivo, which means "outside the body," describes
gene therapy procedures in which damaged cells are
removed from a patient, treated, and then returned
to the patient's body. In the treatment, viral vectors
are used to transport new, healthy DNA *(red)* into
the patient's cells, where it joins with the cell's
existing DNA *(yellow)*. In the case of Ashi DeSilva,
the new DNA told her cells to produce an enzyme
that her body had not been making on its own.

From 1990 to 1992, Ashi received ten more follow-up gene therapy treatments to make sure that an even greater number of her white blood cells had healthy *ADA* genes. She was also given regular injections of the ADA enzyme for extra safety. The doctors wanted to do everything possible to make sure that her immune system stayed strong.

More than ten years after her treatment, Ashi is still doing well. She still receives the ADA enzyme on a regular basis, but her immune system remains strong. In fact, it's significantly stronger than the immune systems of patients receiving injections of the ADA enzyme who have not been through gene therapy. According to W. French Anderson, one of Ashi's doctors, this success story proves that "if you put a correct gene into enough cells in a patient, you will correct the disease."

A ROLLER COASTER RIDE

Gene therapy is a promising technology. Ashanthi DeSilva's success was a high point for researchers. Since then, one-quarter of the world's SCID patients have benefited from SCID gene therapy. One patient, Rhys Evans from Wales, United Kingdom, suffering from a slightly different form of SCID, was cured entirely when he was eighteen months old. Rhys has a healthy immune system, and he does not need to take any extra enzymes to make sure that he stays healthy. According to Rhys's mother, gene therapy is "nothing short of a miracle."

Unfortunately, gene therapy has had some low points too. In 1999 Jesse Gelsinger, an eighteen-year-old with a mild enzyme disorder, volunteered to undergo gene therapy. Jesse did not have a life-threatening disease, but he knew that some young children had a more serious form of his disorder. Jesse wanted to help

Free from the confines of their hospital rooms, Ashi DeSilva *(far right)* sits with another SCID patient, Cynthia Cutshall. Dr. W. French Anderson treated the girls with gene therapy in the early 1990s.

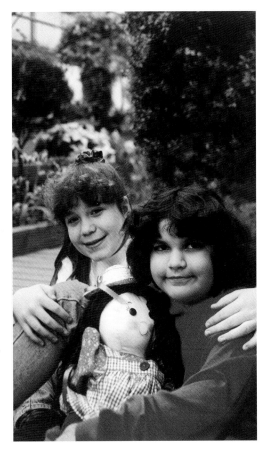

these patients, so he agreed to test a new gene therapy procedure designed to cure the disease.

When doctors injected Jesse with a heavy dose of genetically altered cold-virus vectors, his body recognized them as invaders. Because the dose was so great, Jesse's immune system went into overdrive. He developed a fever, then lapsed into a coma. Finally, his entire body shut down. Doctors could do nothing to save him. Within four days of receiving the vectors, Jesse Gelsinger was dead.

The doctors overseeing the gene therapy trial had been in a hurry to test their technique. They needed to prove that it worked in humans. Then they could get U.S. Food and Drug Administration (FDA) approval and begin selling it for profit.

In their haste, the doctors failed to tell Jesse and his parents about problems with earlier trials. Two rhesus monkeys treated with the same technique had died, and four human subjects had suffered liver damage. When the FDA reviewed the case, they said the doctors never should have tested the technique on Jesse Gelsinger—or on anyone else. Jesse Gelsinger's death made medical researchers think twice about their methods.

Gene therapy suffered another blow in 2002. In France two young boys with SCID underwent a procedure similar to Ashanthi DeSilva's. But instead of behaving normally and repairing their immune system, their white blood cells started multiplying out of control. The result was leukemia, a life-threatening cancer of the blood. Scientists strongly suspect that the gene therapy was responsible for the leukemia. Even though both boys' cancer responded well to radiation therapy, scientists remain very concerned about this unexpected result.

Following this failure, the FDA took quick action in the United States. The FDA oversees U.S. application of pioneering medical procedures such as gene therapy. On January 14, 2003, the FDA announced that U.S. scientists could continue with gene therapy trials on animals. A temporary ban, however, was placed on trials that used viral vectors as delivery devices and involved human subjects. The FDA planned to review the situation on an ongoing basis to decide how long the ban should last.

SLOW PROGRESS

After the FDA ban, American scientists limited their gene therapy research to laboratory animals. At universities in Florida and Texas, researchers pursued a cure for Canavan disease, a rare degenerative brain disease. In California another group of scientists studied Alzheimer's, a disease that affects memory. In both projects, gene therapy improved the condition of damaged brain tissue in laboratory mice.

Both of these projects used viral vectors. But as we have seen, viral vector delivery systems can lead to unpredictable and sometimes dangerous results. If viruses are given to a person several times, the immune system may start attacking them. Viruses also may interfere with a cell's natural functioning and may trigger disease, since they must infect the cell to get into it. Researchers at the Carnegie Mellon University in Pennsylvania are developing a new kind of delivery system that they believe will be more predictable and safer than viral vectors. Instead of whole viruses, the Carnegie Mellon researchers' system uses tiny beads called nanoparticles. A nanoparticle is a tiny fragment of a virus. Scientists load healthy genes into the nanoparticles. Then, after the particles enter the nucleus of the target cells, the healthy genes are released. While viral vectors can trigger diseases by delivering their gene payloads to the wrong place in the genome, researchers have found that nanoparticles are more accurate at delivering their payload to the right place.

All of these gene therapy projects are in early experimental stages. No one can say for sure which ones will eventually be offered to the public or when. First, they must be proven safe and effective. Some experts predict that practical gene therapy procedures will be available by 2010. Others say it may take another twenty years. While researchers disagree about the timetable, most are confident that gene therapy techniques will eventually be used to treat and cure a wide range of diseases.

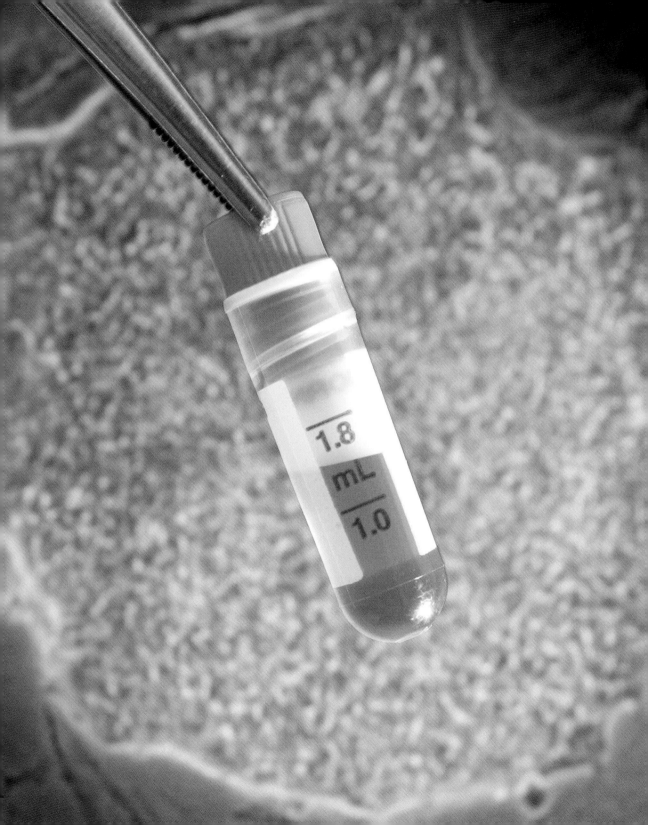

Chapter Four

STEMS AND SNIPS

So far we have looked at somatic gene therapy procedures that repair damage inside the cell. Researchers are also developing another form of gene therapy in which the patient receives brand-new cells to replace cells damaged or killed by disease. Instead of fixing cells that are not working properly, this therapy provides new cells to do the jobs that the existing cells weren't doing.

Where do the brand-new cells come from? They come from stem cells. Most of the cells in your body are specialized: brain cells, lung cells, blood cells, and so forth. Think of all these specialized cells as adults. Each one works at a special kind of job, like teachers, mail carriers, bus drivers, or dentists. Stem cells, on the other hand, have not yet specialized. Think of them as young people who haven't decided what they want to be when they grow up. Until they decide, stem cells have the potential to develop into *any* kind of cell.

Scientists get some stem cells from embryos. In the human reproductive process, a sperm cell fertilizes an egg cell, and the newly created embryo begins dividing. At this point, all the cells that make up the embryo are stem cells. But as the weeks pass, each embryonic stem cell gradually transforms, turning into one particular type of cell. As stem cells transform, so does the embryo.

A small vial containing human stem cells is shown against a background of an enlarged stem cell *(facing page).* **Stem cells have the potential to develop into any type of cell in the body.**

It changes from a blob of identical stem cells to a human fetus with recognizable arms, legs, fingers, toes, and so forth.

Gene therapy researchers get embryonic stem cells from embryos created during in vitro fertilization (IVF) procedures. IVF is a medical procedure for couples who cannot conceive a child by means of sexual intercourse. Scientists use the couple's eggs and sperm to grow embryos in lab dishes. Some of these embryos are transplanted into the woman's uterus to grow into a baby. If the couple chooses to donate their leftover embryos for scientific research, those embryos can supply stem cells for gene therapy trials.

To prepare fetal stem cells for gene therapy procedures, scientists place them in lab dishes and treat them with chemicals and electricity. This coaxes the stem cells to grow into the kind of cells a patient needs. The scientists culture, or grow, copies of these cells in test tubes. Then the cells are ready for transplanting into the patient. Patients with Alzheimer's disease, for example, need new brain tissue to replace the tissue the disease has destroyed. What would happen if scientists could create the right kind of specialized brain cells and successfully insert them into a patient's body? Scientists believe the healthy new cells would continue to grow and divide until they formed healthy new brain tissue to replace the damaged tissue. Gene therapy with fetal stem cells is risky, however, because it involves foreign cells that contain someone else's genome. As a result, they are more likely to be rejected if the patient's immune system recognizes them as invaders.

Scientists can also get stem cells from children and adults. While most of an adult's cells are specialized, the body does contain some stem cells to repair damaged tissue. When you get a cut, stem cells in your skin travel to the injury to develop

A researcher holds a petri dish containing a sample of human stem cells. The cells are growing into specialized cells through the use of chemicals and an incubator *(left)*—a device that provides a controlled atmosphere and encourages growth of microorganisms.

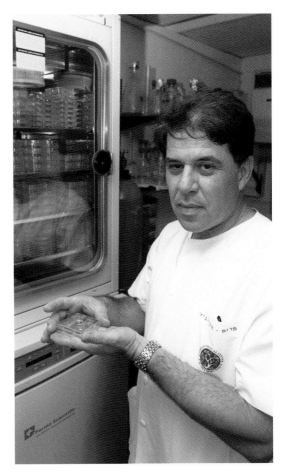

into new skin tissue. But when a serious disease sets in, your body may not be able to make enough stem cells to repair all the damage.

This is where gene therapy might be able to help. If researchers can supply a patient with enough extra stem cells from his or her own body, the patient's body may be able to heal itself. In February 2003, sixteen-year-old Dimitri Bonnville was accidentally shot in the heart with a nail gun at a construction site. A month later, he became the first person in the world to get a stem cell transplant to his heart, using stem cells gathered from his own blood. Doctors transplanted the cells into the artery that supplies blood to the front wall of the heart, where the heart muscle was severely damaged.

Doctors saw immediate improvement. The stem cells appeared to strengthen Dimitri's damaged heart.

Dimitri Bonnville's stem cells were collected directly from his own blood to ensure that his body would not reject the new cells. If the stem cells had not been genetically identical to the rest of his cells, his body probably would have identified the foreign cells as invaders and destroyed them.

Adult stem cells are perfect for gene therapy procedures, but they may also have other important uses. Each day in the United States, eighteen people die while waiting for organ transplants. People who do receive organ transplants may also die if their immune system sees the new organ as an invader and rejects it. In the future, researchers may be able to save these patients by giving them healthy new organs, such as livers and hearts, grown from the patients' own stem cells. Organs grown from stem cells could also be used to prolong lives. As people grow older, their organs begin to wear out. If doctors could replace a person's old organs with new ones grown from that

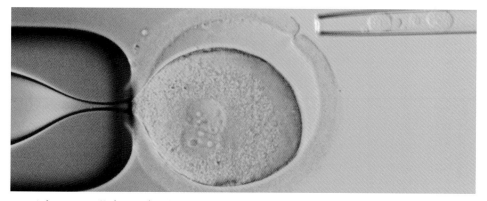

A human cell *(center)* is held in position by a pipette, or suction tool *(left)*, to receive healthy genetic material *(right)* as part of gene therapy.

person's own stem cells, it's possible that more people could live longer and healthier lives.

Extracting adult stem cells can be difficult. To create greater numbers of stem cells that are genetically identical to a patient, scientists are developing a technique called therapeutic cloning. In this technique, scientists begin with a human egg cell, remove its nucleus, and insert the nucleus from a cell belonging to the patient. Then they prompt the egg cell to begin dividing. As the egg cell divides, it creates stem cells.

Like other forms of gene therapy, therapeutic cloning is still in the experimental stage. In nearly all trials, the patient is a test animal, not a human. Still, some trial results seem promising. In 2002 a team of Massachusetts researchers used therapeutic cloning to produce stem cells to repair a mouse's damaged immune system. Their success suggests that therapeutic cloning could work on humans someday. That's good news, since therapeutic cloning is potentially safer than other forms of gene therapy because it doesn't risk rejection.

But before scientists can even consider human trials, they will have to move beyond mice and try therapeutic cloning on more complex animals, such as monkeys. According to Robert Lanza, who conducts therapeutic cloning research at Advanced Cell Technology in Worcester, Massachusetts, "The real challenge is to get things to work in large animals with sophisticated immune systems similar to a human's." Then it's on to *Homo sapiens*—humans.

SNIPS AND ALLELES

One day, gene therapy may revolutionize the way genetic diseases are treated. Instead of treating the patient's symptoms, doctors would treat the patient's genome. This would be a radical leap forward in medical treatment. As scientists work toward this goal, they are also improving standard medical treatments in small but important ways. The key to these advances lies in the differences between people's genomes.

All human genomes are roughly 99.9 percent alike. Of the genome's three billion nucleotide bases, all but about three million are exactly the same. But this 0.1 percent difference is still highly significant. It makes your genome different from everyone else's.

We all have the same set of genes, but some genes come in different varieties. Scientists call different varieties of the same gene alleles. The differences between alleles are tiny. The average gene has roughly three thousand nucleotide base pairs, and most alleles differ by only one base pair. These single-base differences are known as single nucleotide polymorphisms, or SNPs (pronounced "snips"). Each person has his or her own unique set of SNPs. According to experts, each person's genome contains between three million and ten million SNPs.

SNPs account for obvious physical differences between people, such as hair color and eye color. More important, SNPs affect people's chances of getting certain diseases during their lifetime. Researchers have located some of the SNPs that make a person more likely to get cancer, heart disease, and other genetic disorders. SNPs can also affect how a patient responds to prescription drugs and other medical treatments.

Currently, doctors prescribe drugs to treat genetic diseases on a hit-and-miss basis. They have a good idea of how a given drug affects people in general, but they can't be certain how it will affect any one particular patient. Since SNPs can affect a patient's response to medications, a drug that works well for one patient might not work well for another patient with the same disease.

"There may be as many as one hundred thousand deaths a year in the U.S. due to bad reactions to drugs prescribed to patients," says Northwestern University's Rex Chisholm. "Another 30 to 40 percent of patients don't respond to certain drugs. The drugs don't harm them, but they don't help them either. Many of these deaths and non-responses are due to genetic factors."

In the future, doctors will be able to find out exactly which SNPs a patient has. Then doctors may be able to prescribe just the right combination of drugs or other treatments for that patient. But doctors will not know which SNPs a patient has until they have a complete profile of that patient's genome. That's why doctors look forward to developing a DNA chip that can hold a patient's complete genetic profile.

Genetic profiling holds special promise for cancer patients. So far, doctors have treated these patients according to where their tumors are located—lungs, brain, breast, and so forth. Most patients receive drug therapy (known as chemotherapy), and some also undergo radiation therapy. Both treatments have drawbacks. Radiation therapy kills healthy cells as well as cancerous ones, and both chemotherapy and radiation can cause troublesome side effects such as loss of energy, nausea, and depression.

When doctors have profiles for specific kinds of cancers and for an individual patient, they will be able to prescribe the best kind of treatment for that patient. Researchers are highly optimistic about this kind of personalized medicine. "As we understand more about the genetic basis of specific diseases, we'll be able to design drugs to target the specific genes that cause those diseases," says Chisholm. "That has incredible potential."

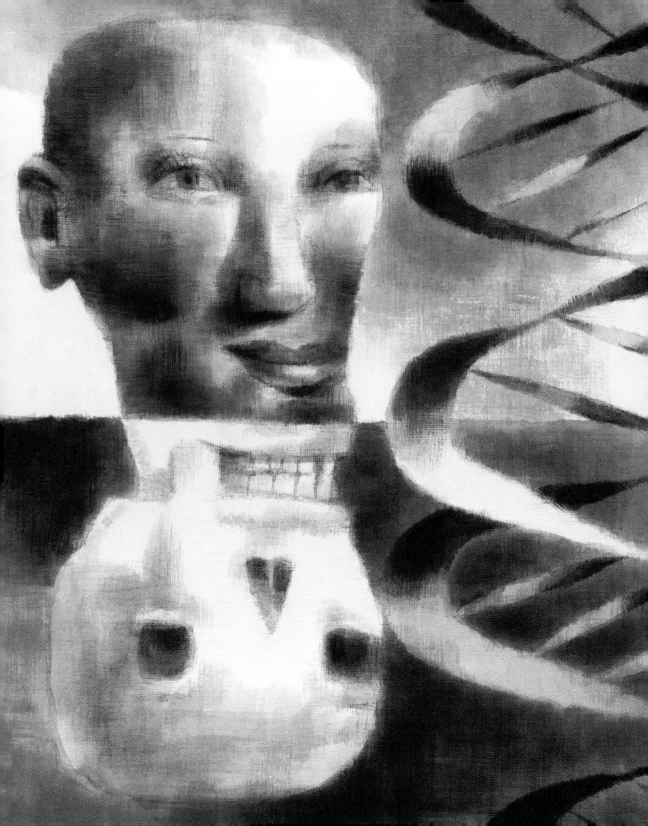

Chapter Five

LIVING LONGER

In addition to promising a healthier life, the genomic revolution holds the possibility of a longer life. Genomic researchers tackle aging in the same way that they go after diseases. First, they work to find the causes. Then they look for ways to counteract them.

As people age, the systems that keep their bodies running gradually break down. Over the years, the muscular system breaks down—as do the nervous system and the respiratory system and so on. The older a person gets, the more these vital systems tend to deteriorate.

Why don't our muscles and nerves and lungs keep on working forever? Experts say the answer lies hidden in our genes. Our genes, like those of all living things, are designed to help our species survive. For a species to survive over hundreds, thousands, even millions of years, each generation of adults must produce a new generation of young.

The human body is designed to produce children until about the age of forty. After that, an adult's most important biological role is caring for children. As far as nature is concerned, by the time adult humans reach the age of fifty-five, their children can live on their own and these adults are no longer needed for the species to survive. That's why so many people begin to have

This illustration (*facing page*) **shows an artist's depiction of the link between increasing genetic knowledge and the potential for increased life span and improved quality of life.**

health problems at around this age. The mutations that have been accumulating in their genes since birth begin to take their toll. Eventually, critical body systems break down completely and people die.

Aging may be a natural process, but that doesn't mean we can't slow it down. Eating a balanced diet and exercising regularly can help us live longer. So can avoiding smoking, drinking alcohol, and breathing exhaust fumes. But even if we do everything humanly possible to stay healthy, we still can't stop our bodies from aging. After all, we can't prevent our genes from mutating. At least we can't yet. But someday that may change.

TELOMERES AND AGING

As scientists learn more about the human genome, they hope to discover strategies for counteracting the genetic causes of aging. For that reason, some scientists are studying telomeres—stretches of DNA at the tips of chromosomes. The nucleotide bases that make up telomeres repeat the same six-letter "junk DNA" sequence—TTAGGG—thousands of times. Even though telomeres do not contain genes, they are vitally important to keeping genes healthy. Like the plastic tips on shoelaces, they protect the ends of chromosomes from wear and tear.

When DNA replicates just before cell division, the copying does not begin right at the tip of a chromosome. As a result, a little bit of the DNA at the end of the chromosome is snipped off. If the missing nucleotides were part of a gene, the new DNA copy would be missing vital information. But since the telomere is made of "junk" DNA, a bit of that gets left out instead, and things go on normally.

In the short run, that's good news. But over time, telomeres keep getting snipped and snipped, becoming shorter and shorter. Finally, after the DNA has copied itself about fifty times, the telomere's "junk" sequence is all used up. Then the chromosome is like a shoelace without the plastic tips. At this point, the cell stops dividing and dies. When a critical number of cells in a part of the body—the liver, for example—die, then the liver can't do its job as well as it did when the person was younger.

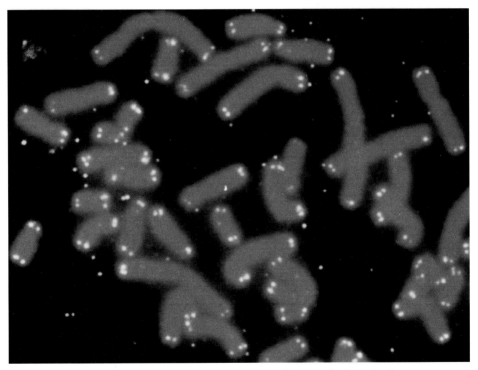

Stained chromosomes reveal telomeres at their tips *(yellow dots)*.
The telomeres protect chromosomes and their vital genetic information from wear and tear. Scientists believe that the eventual breakdown of telomeres may be one cause of aging.

Some scientists think that if telomeres could be repaired or resupplied, genes could be protected and new cells would keep on doing their jobs. How could researchers trick the body into rebuilding telomeres? The answer may lie in telomerase, an enzyme that maintains telomeres in stem cells. In nearly all adult cells, the genes that code for telomerase are permanently turned off. If researchers could find a way to switch telomerase genes back on, telomeres in adult cells could be maintained and many more generations of new cells would have all the genes they needed to go on working properly.

The result would be a longer, healthier life. But that doesn't mean we could go on living forever. Wear and tear of telomeres is only one of the reasons our bodies age and die. Still, scientists hope that we will eventually be able to control the activity of telomerase in heart cells, brain cells, and other vital adult cells.

VANDALS AND OVERACHIEVERS

Other researchers are trying to prolong life by different means. Some work with molecules known as free radicals. These molecules are called *free* because they have no set job to do—they are free to roam about the genome. They can damage the mechanisms cells use to copy and repair themselves. Free radicals are a bit like people out to make trouble. That's why some scientists have nicknamed them the vandals of the genome.

The damage caused by free radicals, like other mutations, accumulates over the years. Experts think the accumulated damage from free radicals is a major cause of aging. It can disrupt DNA replication and cause mutations that trigger age-related diseases such as heart disease and some forms of cancer.

While some scientists are busy searching for ways to control free radicals, others are studying the genome of centenarians— people who are at least one hundred years old. Thomas Perls, a researcher at Boston University School of Medicine in Boston, Massachusetts, directed one of these studies. He and his research team discovered that some centenarians had ignored the rules of healthy living. They had smoked cigarettes, eaten lots of fatty foods and few fresh fruits and vegetables, or exercised very little during their long lives. Yet they had been ill less than most of the people who never smoke, who eat healthful diets, and who exercise on a regular basis.

How could this be? Did these centenarians carry special superyouth genes? Not necessarily. Perls and his team suspect that the centenarians may have the same genes as everyone else, but that some of the genes are superactive. In other words, genes related to fighting disease may stay switched on more of the time than in ordinary people. This would explain why centenarians tend to get sick less often throughout their lives. Scientists have a special name for these genes related to long life. Since *longevity* means "long life," they call them longevity genes.

Using genotyping, Perls and his team have determined that a section of chromosome 4 is highly likely to have a number of longevity genes. Other research teams are looking for more of these superactive genes in other parts of the genome. Meanwhile, still other teams are trying to find out what keeps these genes switched on for such long periods of time in the centenarians. Their goal is to learn how to keep longevity genes activated in everyone's genomes, so that someday we may all live longer, healthier lives.

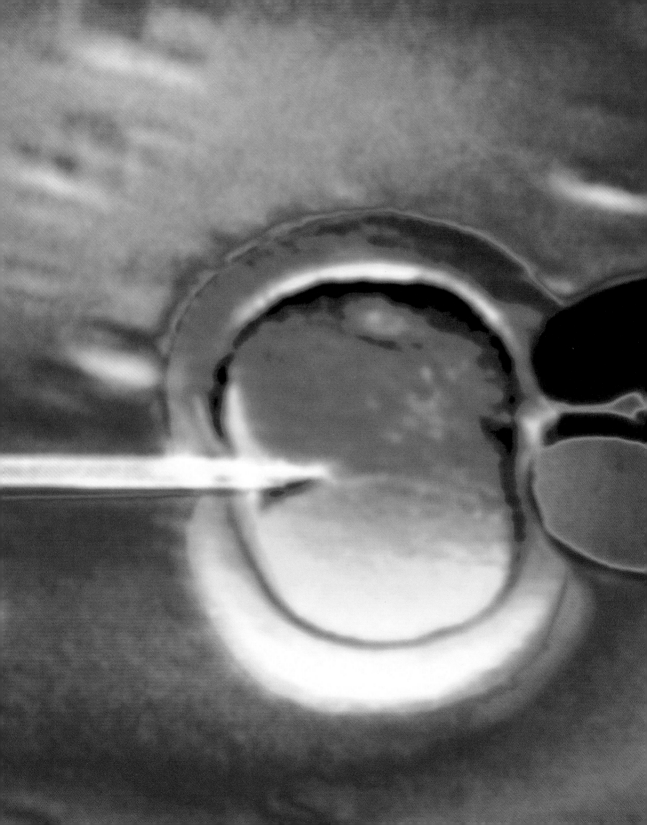

Chapter Six

ENGINEERING OURSELVES

The new knowledge generated by the Human Genome Project will likely help scientists and doctors conquer illness and lengthen life. In addition, it holds the promise of creating more perfect genomes. How perfect? Let's start with children. Some scientists foresee a day when parents may have their babies carefully designed in a laboratory, gene by gene.

Scientists weren't thinking about designing babies' genomes when they developed in vitro fertilization. Still, an important part of the IVF process has helped to pave the way for designer babies.

In IVF, an egg cell is fertilized in a lab dish to create an embryo. Then the embryo is implanted in the mother's uterus to develop into a baby. Before implantation, scientists carefully screen, or examine, the embryo's genome to make sure it's healthy. This screening process is known as preimplantation genetic diagnosis (PGD).

PGD screening is especially vital when one or both parents carry damaged genes that could lead to serious single-gene disorders, such as some forms of Alzheimer's or Huntington's disease. Because genes are inherited, or passed from parent to child, some IVF embryos carry the same damaged genes as their parents' genomes carry. PGD allows doctors to ensure that only embryos with healthy genes are chosen for implantation.

Thermal (heat) photography highlights a human egg cell (*facing page, center*) **being fertilized with sperm** (*facing page, left*) **in a process known as in vitro fertilization.**

In 1999 a thirty-year-old Chicago woman decided that she wanted to have a baby. She knew she had a mutated gene that made her likely to develop a rare and severe form of Alzheimer's disease, and she wanted to be sure her baby would not inherit this mutation. IVF and PGD were the perfect solution. After her egg cells were mixed with her husband's sperm cells to create embryos, the woman's doctor used PGD to identify an embryo free of the Alzheimer's mutation. This healthy embryo was implanted in her uterus, and nine months later, she gave birth to a healthy baby girl whose genome was free of the Alzheimer's mutation.

Doctors currently use PGD for one reason only—to produce healthy babies. But the day may come when scientists can use an advanced version of this procedure to analyze an embryo's entire genome. Then, using other new techniques, scientists might be able to alter some of the genes for reasons other than health.

Genes come in different alleles (varieties). Using gene therapy, scientists could swap alleles in an embryo to produce a baby with a genome chosen by the parents. Some of the alleles might be selected to improve the baby's health—but others might give a child a certain appearance, a certain personality, and a certain set of talents. The parents' goal would be to design the most perfect child possible.

Will it ever become possible to fine-tune a genome so precisely? Science author Matt Ridley considers the possibility: "As the third millennium dawns," he writes, "we are for the first time in a position to edit the text of our genetic code. . . . We can cut bits out, add bits in, rearrange paragraphs or write over words."

If designing a child's genome ever becomes possible, the process might go something like this. First, the parents-to-be decide whether they want to have a boy or a girl. Then they study a chart that lists various alleles, that describes the effect each allele has, and that gives the cost of engineering each allele into a child's genome.

Using the chart, the parents-to-be choose alleles that will give their child a certain physical appearance. They choose a certain shape and color for the eyes. They choose alleles for their child's height and weight, and the color and thickness of hair. Do they want their child to have freckles or dimples? There are alleles they can choose for these features. They also choose alleles for the shape and prominence of the nose, cheek-bones, and chin. And so on.

Next, these designing parents select genes that will influence their child's talents and behavior. They might pick alleles that tend to make the child a skilled musician or mathematician or basketball player. They might choose alleles that tend to cause positive behavior traits, such as ambition, self-confidence, or optimism. In short, these parents-to-be design a genetic profile for the most perfect child they can imagine. Then doctors use IVF and gene therapy techniques to create the "perfect" child the parents want.

COULD WE? SHOULD WE?

Will designer babies ever become reality? The idea may sound like pure science fiction, but not long ago, many people said the same thing about such procedures as IVF and PGD. Since 1978, when the first IVF baby was born, the procedure has become more and more common at hospitals worldwide. To date, an estimated seven hundred healthy babies have been born worldwide to parents who used both IVF and PGD.

Like IVF and PGD, designer babies may eventually become science fact. But first, scientists must develop safe and effective gene therapy techniques to edit the genome precisely. Then they must locate all the genes that influence appearance, talents, and behavior. In most cases, a complex network of genes is involved, so researchers must also learn exactly how these networks operate.

How close are scientists to achieving these goals? They have already identified alleles that code for eye and hair color. As researchers learn more about the genome, they will discover alleles for other physical features. Some experts are confident that gene therapy will one day be used to design a child's outward appearance.

They are much less confident about talents and behavior. Researchers have used genotyping to locate a few genes that appear to influence these traits. What would happen if they could locate all the genes involved and learn how they all work together? Most experts agree that even then, no one in any laboratory could ever "design" a great pianist or mathematician or soccer player. They feel the same way about behavioral traits such as self-confidence and optimism. Genes may be part of the recipe for talent and behavior, but many other ingredients also have an influence. Nutrition, environment, upbringing, and the influence of friends all play important roles in developing a person's talents and behavior.

For a moment, though, let's suppose scientists could "design" a person in the laboratory, choosing appearance, talents, and behavior. Should they? Many researchers say no, and many political and religious leaders agree. They believe that genetically designing people would be morally and ethically wrong. Any attempt to "perfect" the human genome would be a disaster for the human race, they insist.

Genetic researchers with humanized mice. The mice genomes have been altered to contain human genetic material. For safety and ethical reasons, scientists conduct nearly all genetic experiments with animals rather than humans.

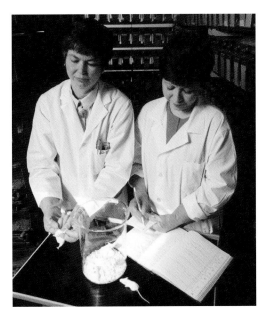

CLONING HUMANS

While some scientists work toward the goal of designing "perfect" people, others are busy developing ways to make perfect copies of people who already exist. These researchers want to clone human beings. Some scientists have already cloned several other mammal species, as described in chapter 9.

Like designer babies, human clones are still science fiction. But let's pretend a human clone does exist—a male named Steve. To create Steve, scientists went through a process known as reproductive cloning. First, they obtained an unfertilized egg from an anonymous female donor. Then they removed the nucleus from the donor's egg cell and replaced it with the nucleus from a cell belonging to Steve's "parent." We'll call him Michael. The nucleus from Michael's cell contains his entire genome.

CELL DONOR (PERSON TO BE CLONED)

HUMAN EGG DONOR

DONOR BODY CELL

DONOR EGG

ENUCLEATION (REMOVAL OF BODY CELL NUCLEUS)

ENUCLEATION (REMOVAL OF EGG CELL NUCLEUS)

ADULT BODY CELL NUCLEUS FUSED INTO DONOR EGG CELL WITH ELECTRICITY

EMBRYO IMPLANTED INTO SURROGATE MOTHER'S UTERUS

HUMAN REPRODUCTIVE CLONING

In human reproductive cloning, the nucleus from an adult body cell would be fused with an enucleated egg to create an embryo. The genome of the embryo would be identical to the genome of the person who donated the adult body cell. The embryo would be implanted into the uterus of a surrogate mother and develop into a baby. This result is called a clone.

NINE MONTHS LATER, CLONED BABY IS BORN

After the nucleus was inserted into the egg cell, scientists stimulated the egg to make it divide and grow. After a few weeks, the resulting embryo was implanted into the uterus of a surrogate, or substitute, mother. Nine months later, Michael's son and clone, Steve, was born.

Let's say that several years have passed, and Steve has a playmate, Jimmy, who was not cloned. What makes Steve and Jimmy different? The difference lies in their genomes. Jimmy's genome is a combination of genes from his two parents' genomes, but Steve has only one genetic parent. Steve's cloned genome is virtually identical to Michael's. People already notice how much young Steve resembles his father. As Steve grows older, the resemblance will grow too. Why? Because, in a way, Michael and Steve are more than father and son. They are also identical twins.

This kind of relationship might seem like a very strange idea, but some experts believe that cloned humans will eventually become science fact. Why would someone want a clone of himself or herself? Here are some reasons.

- Female couples who did not want to undergo IVF with sperm from a male donor could have a child on their own. One woman could provide the unfertilized egg. The other could supply the donor DNA. Then either woman could be the birth mother and carry the baby until it was born.

- Single people without partners might want a child born with their genome only. A single woman could provide both the unfertilized egg and the donor DNA, and then give birth herself. A single man, like Michael in the example above, would need to find a surrogate mother and a woman willing to donate an unfertilized egg.

After the single man's DNA is inserted into the donor egg, the surrogate mother would carry the baby until it was born.

- A couple whose child has died in an accident could have the child cloned. They would use an unfertilized egg from the mother and donor DNA saved from the deceased child.

While human cloning may someday be possible, that doesn't make it a good idea. A great many people have strong moral or ethical objections to cloning humans.

ENHANCING GENOMES

Another promise of the genomic revolution is genetic enhancement, or improvement. Genetic enhancement is still just an idea, a potential goal. But like designer babies and human cloning, it may one day be a reality.

Here's how it would work. Let's say there are qualities about yourself that you'd like to change. Maybe you're going bald, and you'd rather have a full head of hair. Maybe you think you're too nervous or not smart enough or too shy. To get back your hair and become calmer or more intelligent or more outgoing, all you'd have to do is go to your doctor for gene therapy. During each treatment, the doctor would add new, improved alleles to your genome. After a few doses, you'd begin to see your hair and your personality transformed. Soon you'd be a new, improved version of yourself.

Before genetic enhancement can ever become possible, scientists will have to learn a great deal more about the genome. First, they will have to locate the networks of genes responsible for the qualities you want enhanced and figure out how these networks operate. They will also have to develop safe, effective gene therapy techniques in order to add the new alleles to your genome.

Some experts doubt that scientists will accomplish these goals anytime soon, if ever. Others insist that, while it may take a decade or two, genetic enhancement will become a reality—though perhaps a very expensive reality. But even if we have the ability to enhance our genomes, an important question still remains: should we?

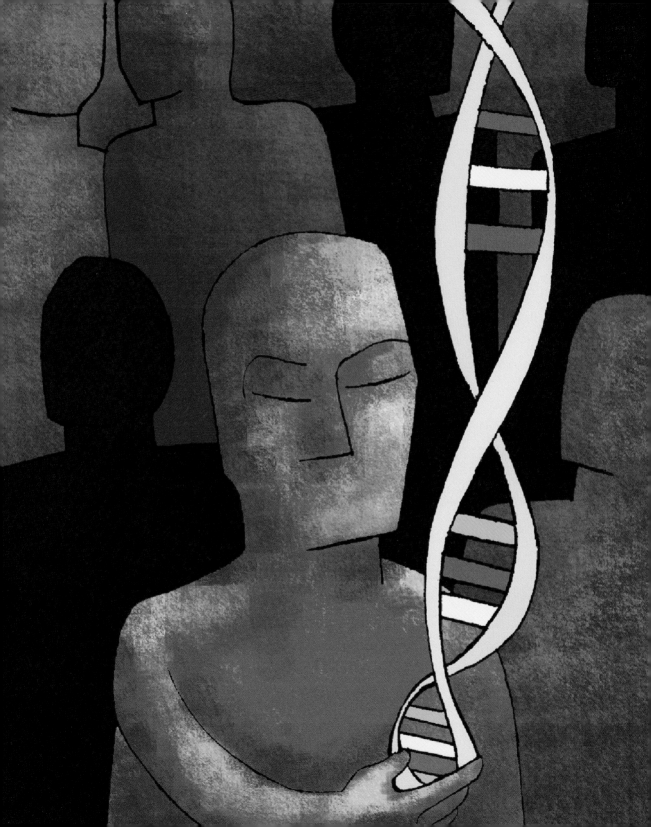

Chapter Seven

HOW FAR SHOULD WE GO?

The potential benefits of the genomic revolution sound wonderful. Who could argue against better health and longer life? But with these benefits come a number of potential perils. In some cases, even the scientists doing the research have concerns about how new knowledge and techniques will be used.

Many researchers worry about the safety of patients. They say we do not know enough about gene therapy to use it safely on human beings. As evidence, they point to doctors' poor judgment in using gene therapy on Jesse Gelsinger. Following Jesse's tragic death, Francis Collins, head of the HGP and director of the National Human Genome Research Institute in Bethesda, Maryland, said, "We had considered gene therapy, I think, unrealistically, as an approach which had enormous promise and very low risk. . . . [T]he notion that gene therapy was entirely safe, compared to other approaches, went out the window with the death of this young man."

Although a great deal more research is needed, some experts believe that the day will come when gene therapy is safe and effective enough to use on a regular basis. But others wonder if we can ever truly understand all the risks involved in altering human genomes. Just because we have the know-how to manipulate genes doesn't mean we should do it, they insist.

The painting on the facing page depicts the idea that for the first time in history, humans have the power to control and change their genomes. Not all people agree that using this power will lead to greater good.

In their book *The Terrible Gift: The Brave New World of Genetic Medicine,* genetic experts Rick J. Carlson and Gary Stimeling warn, "[W]e're children playing with really big matches."

GERMLINE ENGINEERING

Scientists' doubts and fears about engineering human genomes are strongest when it comes to germline engineering—also called germline therapy. In the future, designer babies could be products of germline engineering. In germline engineering, scientists make changes to the egg and sperm cells, also known as germ cells. These changes are permanent. They would be copied into every cell of the baby created with the modified egg and sperm cells. In addition, these changes would become part of the genome of every one of that person's children and grandchildren for all the generations to come.

Germline engineering is officially outlawed in Germany and parts of Europe. While it is not officially illegal in the United States, polls show that a great many Americans would like to see it outlawed.

Why are so many people opposed to germline engineering? One big reason is eugenics, a social movement that first became popular during the late 1800s in Europe and the United States. Supporters of eugenics started out with good intentions. They wanted to make the whole human race healthier and smarter. But the methods they used to reach this goal turned their good intentions into a catastrophe for the human race.

At first, supporters of eugenics urged people who were mentally and physically fit to have lots of children. Then they asked lawmakers to find ways to prevent other people from having any children. These "others" included African Americans,

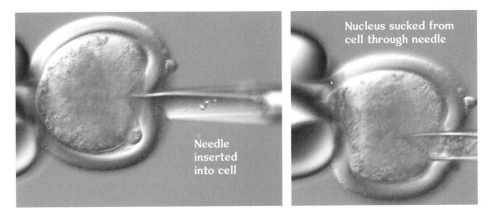

In the process of enucleation *(above)*, the nucleus of an egg cell
is carefully removed with a fine needle, keeping the cell intact.
Enucleation makes the next step of germline engineering
possible—the insertion of a genome-enhanced nucleus.

people who were mentally ill, and people who had committed
violent crimes. In the United States, some states passed laws
allowing doctors to sterilize these "unfit" people.

Many Americans, including President Theodore Roosevelt,
agreed with these laws. Roosevelt told Americans that "the
prime duty, the inescapable duty, of the good citizen of the
right type is to leave his or her blood behind him in the world."
U.S. Supreme Court justice Oliver Wendell Holmes was more
blunt: "We want people who are healthy, good-natured, emo-
tionally stable, sympathetic, and smart. We do not want idiots,
imbeciles, paupers, and criminals."

An estimated 60,000 to 100,000 people in the United States
were sterilized against their will before the eugenics movement
came to an end. The movement began losing popularity
in the United States during the 1930s. During that decade,
Adolf Hitler and his Nazi Party came to power in Germany,

and Hitler declared entire races of people unwanted and unfit to live. The end result was the Holocaust—the horrific murder of many people, including about six million Jewish people. The Holocaust demonstrated that the ideas behind the eugenics movement could lead to unimaginable horrors.

The eugenics movement took place long before germline engineering was possible, but the two have a similar goal—to enhance the human race by improving people's genetic makeup. That's why many people have serious doubts about germline engineering. They worry that new genetic technology might lead to the development of a superrace like the one Hitler had in mind. Author Francis Fukuyama writes, "Human genetic engineering raises most directly the prospect of a new kind of eugenics, with all the moral implications with which the word is fraught, and ultimately the power to change human nature."

It may be years before scientists test germline engineering techniques on human subjects, but people aren't waiting to voice their concerns. David King is a genetic researcher who founded the Campaign Against Human Genetic Engineering. He says, "We've all known the day would come when we'd have to decide whether or not to allow the reconfiguration of human beings through genetic technology. Well, that day is now."

As the debate on germline engineering heats up, opponents and supporters take their stands on the issues involved. Let's see what each side has to say.

RISK

Opponents of germline engineering argue that the human genome is an incredibly complex and delicate living thing. Our genomes have evolved over millions of years. Germline engineering would alter the human genome in the blink of an eye. No matter how much careful testing researchers do, the risk of unintended consequences remains. Scientists might accidentally create new genes they can't control. Genetically engineered children might not turn out the way we expect. According to opponents, we can't afford to tinker around with the genomes of the next generation of children. That's why they think germline engineering should be banned.

Supporters agree that there are dangers. They admit that scientists will most likely make some mistakes along the way. But, they say, researchers will learn from their mistakes and continue to move forward. Supporters also point out that if germline engineering were banned in the United States, scientists would just move elsewhere to continue their work.

EQUALITY

The Declaration of Independence states that "all men are created equal." This statement is the foundation of democracy. Opponents say that germline engineering would undermine this foundation. Since the procedures would be very expensive, only wealthy people could afford to have their children engineered to be healthier, more talented, and more intelligent. According to opponents, this would lead to a society divided into two distinct classes—the gene-rich and the gene-poor. The gene-rich would make up the privileged class. They would be the commanders, the managers, the executives, the bankers, and the lawmakers. These gene-rich people would pass on their enriched genomes to their children, who would pass them on to theirs.

Meanwhile, the rest of society would continue to pass on their ordinary genes to their children. These gene-poor people would be less healthy, less intelligent, and less powerful. They would spend their lives working for the gene-rich at low-paying jobs. They would become a permanent genetic underclass. Gene-ism would join racism as a form of discrimination.

Supporters of germline engineering point out that "all men are created equal" refers to equal rights. Enhancing genomes would not deny equal rights to anyone, they say. Everyone would still have equal rights under the law.

Nevertheless, supporters are concerned about what might happen if enhancements were available only to wealthy nations and individuals. They admit that this might make the rich richer and the poor poorer and ultimately lead to genetic discrimination. Supporters say that we must remain aware of these potential problems and be prepared to deal with them when human genetic engineering becomes a reality.

PLAYING GOD

Opponents point out that germline engineering would change the nature of human reproduction. Having a baby would no longer be a natural process. Instead, it would be a controlled process, with us in control. We would be playing God, say opponents, and playing God is both physically dangerous and morally wrong. Opponents insist that we should not be tinkering with the creation of human life.

Supporters argue that humans are natural tinkerers. We have always examined the inner workings of things and looked for ways to make them work better. We have always changed things. We have cleared forests for farmland to feed ourselves. We have altered almost everything "natural" on the planet, from deserts to oceans to the air we breathe—all to suit our needs.

Why stop here? supporters ask. Since we have unlocked the secrets of the human genome, why not take control of our own evolution, as we have taken control of everything else on the planet? Lee Silver is a geneticist at Princeton University in Princeton, New Jersey. He writes, "Human beings now have the power not only to control but to create new genes for themselves. Why not seize this power? Why not control what has been left to chance in the past?"

HUMAN RIGHTS

Opponents argue that human genetic engineering would rob children of the most basic human right. Children have the right to design their own selves as they grow into adults. They have the right to become the person *they* choose to be. According to opponents, designer babies would not have this right. Their personalities and talents would already be designed for them.

Supporters argue that parents already mold and shape their children. They give them piano and art lessons. They encourage them to play sports. In some cases, they give them powerful drugs, such as Ritalin and Prozac, to control their behavior and their moods. Geneticist Lee Silver writes, "On what basis can we reject positive genetic influences on a person's essence when we accept the rights of parents to benefit their children in every other way?"

THE HUMAN CLONING DEBATE

No part of the genomic revolution inspires as much opposition as human reproductive cloning. In 2004 researchers from South Korea became the first scientists to clone a human embryo.

They did not attempt to implant the embryo in a woman's uterus to create a human clone, though. They cloned the embryo only to produce stem cells for therapeutic cloning research. One of the researchers, Shin Yong Moon of Seoul National University, said, "Our inspiration is to treat incurable diseases. As scientists, we believe that this study is our responsibility and moral obligation."

Nevertheless, their success stirred up a firestorm of controversy. Critics warned that if this kind of therapeutic cloning is permitted, so-called rogue scientists will be encouraged to move on to the next step and clone humans.

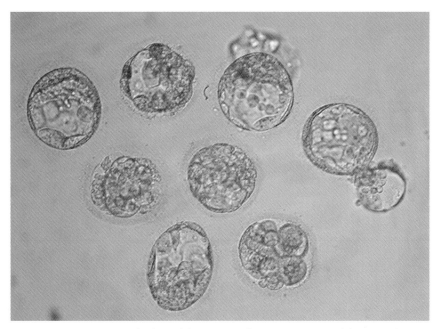

A microscopic view of cloned human embryos generated by South Korean scientists in 2004. The controversial embryos were grown to generate stem cells for scientific research.

No government in the world actively supports human repro-ductive cloning. The government of South Korea prohibits it but provides funds for the kind of therapeutic cloning research conducted by Shin Yong Moon's group. Some nations, such as Germany, have banned all research that involves cloning human embryos, and the United Nations has drafted a treaty to ban human reproductive cloning worldwide. Some world leaders have been outspoken opponents of human reproductive cloning. Former U.S. president Gerald Ford has called human cloning "a perversion of science," and the European Parliament has labeled it "a grave violation of fundamental rights. . . ."

How do U.S. citizens feel about this issue? In a 1997 *Time* magazine/CNN poll, Americans were asked the question, "Is it against God's will to clone human beings?" Of the 1,005 people who responded, 74 percent of them answered yes.

Opponents of human reproductive cloning include promi-nent religious leaders. The Vatican, home of the pope and the Roman Catholic Church, issued a statement calling reproduc-tive cloning a "venture into a tunnel of madness." According to one Catholic priest, "Cloning would only produce humanoids or androids—soulless replicas of human beings."

Supporters of human reproductive cloning argue that these objections are based on myths, not facts. Among these myths is the false belief that a human clone would be an identical copy of its parent, with an identical personality and interests. These clones would have no opportunity to develop their own sense of self, the myth says. They would not be true individuals.

Supporters point out that clones are simply later-born identical twins. Anyone who has ever known identical twins knows that each twin is a distinct individual. Like ordinary identical twins, clones would be free to develop their own unique personalities and interests. They would not be replicas. They would be as much individuals and as independent as anyone else.

TAKING LIFE

Nearly as controversial as human cloning is research that involves embryonic stem cells. Most stem cells used in research come from embryos left over from IVF procedures. Those who oppose this procedure base their objections on moral concerns, with antiabortion groups leading the way. Opponents believe that each person has a sacred soul and that this soul lives in each human cell, even if those cells are in an embryo in a laboratory dish. They also argue that each embryonic stem cell has the capacity to develop into a fully formed human being. Therefore, using these cells for research purposes destroys potential human life. It is the same as murder.

A 2002 report from the President's Council on Bioethics states: "As much as we wish to alleviate suffering now and to leave our children a world where suffering can be more effectively relieved, we also want to leave them a world . . . that honors moral limits, that respects all life whether strong or weak, and that refuses to secure the good of some human beings by sacrificing . . . others."

Supporters of embryonic stem cell research disagree. They argue that stem cells come from discarded embryos. And while these cells are technically alive, they have no organs or central nervous system. They cannot suffer or feel pain, and while these embryos have the potential to become living human beings, they never will. Why throw them away when researchers can use them to help conquer illness? A *Washington Post* editorial in support of therapeutic cloning states: "To use cloned [stem] cells to save lives is not destroying human beings in the service of research. As science evolves, law will have to also. . . . Therapeutic cloning, and the promise it holds for people, should be allowed to proceed, with careful attention to where it goes."

WHAT LAWMAKERS SAY

In the United States, the lion's share of funds for scientific research comes from the federal government. Funding scientific research is a tricky balancing act. Before lawmakers approve money for research, they must carefully consider the opinions of both supporters and opponents of that research. Federal funding for embryonic stem cell research is especially controversial. Opponents insist that this research destroys potential human beings. Supporters point out the potential benefits for conquering disease and relieving human suffering.

In August 2001, President George W. Bush issued a balanced order permitting federal funding for certain kinds of stem cell research, but not for others. He also has made it known that he personally opposes all cloning research, including therapeutic cloning for the purpose of treating diseases.

In 2002 President Bush said: "Human cloning is deeply troubling to me, and to most Americans. . . . Allowing cloning would be taking a significant step toward a society in which human beings are grown for spare body parts, and children are engineered to custom specifications; and that's not acceptable."

In 2003 eleven U.S. senators introduced a bill to ban human reproductive cloning and to permit therapeutic cloning research. The bill died in committee, but lawmakers will continue to debate funding for stem cell research, therapeutic cloning, and other forms of genetic research in the years to come.

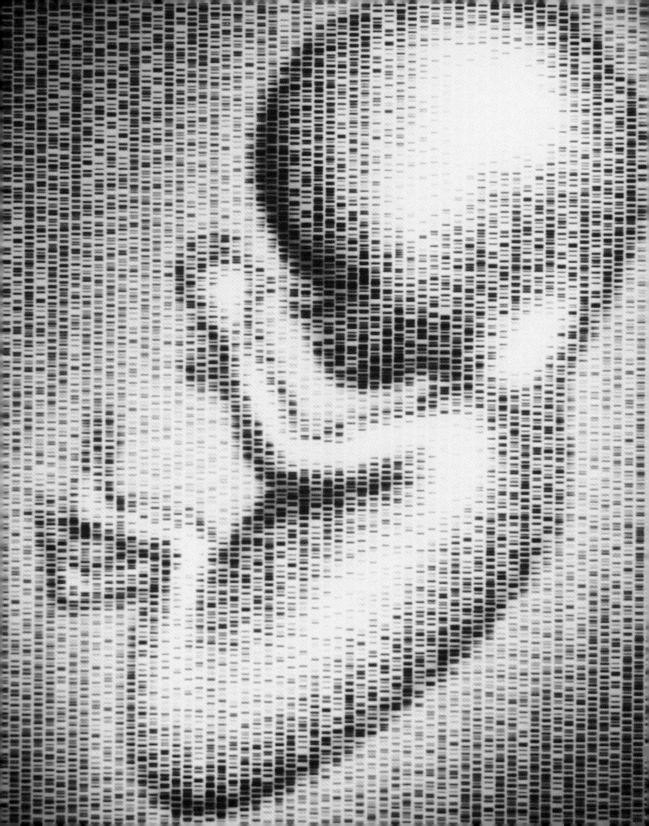

Chapter Eight

PRIVACY AND JUSTICE

Knowing more about the human genome should improve public health, but this knowledge also raises public concerns. Institutions are collecting DNA from more people every day. Hospitals often collect and catalogue DNA samples from newborn children. The U.S. armed forces does the same for all its members. Scientists collect DNA samples to use in their research. Doctors may collect samples from patients, which become a routine part of each patient's medical record.

This information is not supposed to be released to the public, but there is always the chance that it will be. Would you want other people to see a record of your DNA? Remember, there is no such thing as a perfect genome. Everyone carries undesirable mutations.

Scientists have already found mutations that indicate whether a person has a greater-than-average chance of developing certain diseases, such as cancer and heart disease. Of course, people with these mutations don't always get the diseases, and some people without them do. Your genes don't entirely determine your fate. They only hint at what might or might not happen someday.

But what if potential employers or insurance companies begin to take genetic testing too seriously? Suppose your

An artist's depiction of a human fetus and genome *(facing page)*. **The collection and use of human genetic information are highly controversial issues.**

genome shows that you have a greater-than-average chance of getting heart disease someday. Let's say you're applying for a job. Would you want your potential employer to know about your genome? Suppose the company decided not to hire you because of it? Insurance companies might refuse to give you health insurance for the same reason. This would be genetic discrimination.

Craig Venter, who was head of Celera, the biotech company involved in sequencing the human genome, believes we need "legislation prohibiting discrimination on the basis of genetic information. It is essential if the biotechnology revolution is to be realized."

Public opinion polls show that most people agree. They think a person's genetic information should not be released without that person's consent. President Bill Clinton shared these concerns. In 2000 he issued an order that prohibited federal agencies from using genetic information as a basis for hiring or firing federal employees. This order does not apply to private, nongovernment employers, though. Some states, such as Oregon, have passed broader laws against genetic discrimination, but many states have not. This is an issue voters and lawmakers will have to confront in the future.

TO KNOW OR NOT TO KNOW

In coming years, scientists will continue developing genetic tests that reveal more and more about our genomes. Genetic testing can already tell us how likely a person is to trigger lung cancer by smoking cigarettes or invite heart disease by eating lots of fatty foods. This kind of testing is known as risk assessment. It's a way of looking at what fate may have in store for us.

If you had a chance to see your risk assessment test results, would you want to see them? Even though mutant genes only hint at possibilities, bad news might turn you into a genetic hypochondriac—a person who lives in a state of constant anxiety, waiting for a disease to strike. On the other hand, knowing the bad news might prompt you to change your lifestyle for the better. You might avoid smoking cigarettes, drinking alcohol to excess, or other activities that could trigger future problems. You might start eating more healthful foods and getting more exercise. To know or not to know—the choice would be yours.

Let's say the risk assessment test is for something more serious, such as a life-threatening inherited disease. For example, based on their family histories, some women are at risk for carrying inherited mutations for breast cancer. These mutations, if they have them, would increase their chances of getting the disease someday. Would they want to be tested for these mutations? Or would they rather not know?

Studies show that 78 percent of women who may carry these mutations would want genetic testing. These women believe in the statement, "Knowledge is power." Those who would test positive would want to undergo drug therapy or surgery to reduce their risk of getting the cancer before it developed.

Is knowledge always power, though? Suppose you know you may have inherited mutations that could cause an incurable disease, but there's nothing you can do to reduce your risk of developing that fatal disease. In this case, you might not want to have genetic testing. One twenty-eight-year-old man who knew he might have the mutant gene for Huntington's disease chose not to be tested, and his wife agreed with the decision.

"My whole attitude on life is that I don't want to know my destiny," she said.

Do you agree with her? As genetic testing becomes more sophisticated, more and more people will have to decide whether they really want to know what their genomes have to say about their future health.

DEVELOPING POWERFUL NEW TOOLS

Medical testing is not the only reason for collecting and analyzing human DNA. It can also be used to bring criminals to justice and to free wrongly convicted people from prison. Virtually every cell in a person's body contains a copy of the genome, and that genome is as unique as the person's fingerprints. In 1984 a British

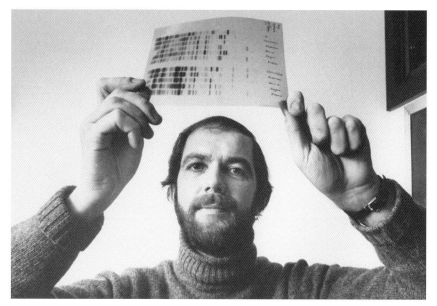

Alec Jeffreys reads a DNA fingerprint, a set of single nucleotide polymorphisms that can be used to genetically identify a person. Jeffreys developed the DNA fingerprinting process in 1984.

Genetic investigators examine human remains found in a mass grave in Bolivia. The investigators will use DNA fingerprinting to help identify the people and to possibly catch their killers.

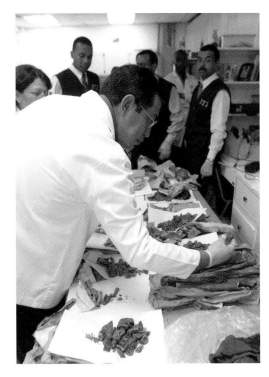

scientist named Alec Jeffreys developed a technique that can be used to identify people from their distinctive genomes. Jeffreys's method is called DNA—or genetic —fingerprinting.

Most of the human genome is identical in all people, but single nucleotide polymorphisms vary from person to person. There can also be even greater variation in "junk DNA" sequences. Jeffreys realized that he could use the unique sequences in a person's "junk DNA" to identify that person.

A few years after developing DNA fingerprinting, Jeffreys used it to analyze DNA evidence in an important criminal case. His test results helped free an innocent man whom police had in custody and to convict the real culprit.

Since then, DNA evidence has helped bring thousands of criminals to justice. It has also liberated people convicted of crimes they didn't commit. Among them are more than one hundred men freed from death row in the United States. Without DNA testing, these innocent men might have been put to death.

PATIENCE VERSUS INSPIRATION

Scientists have all sorts of different personalities. Even though Alec Jeffreys and Kary Mullis made related discoveries at about the same time, their personalities couldn't be more different.

Alec Jeffreys is a patient, methodical researcher who spends most of his time in the laboratory. In the early 1980s, he was trying to separate certain small segments of DNA from the entire genome, make them radioactive, and capture their images on X-ray film. This meticulous, painstaking method took many months to perfect.

Kary Mullis, on the other hand, is an impatient and impulsive researcher. To him, lab work is routine and boring. In the early 1980s, he spent as little time as possible in his northern California laboratory. He preferred to do his research in his head while surfing or driving. One day, while cruising along a highway in his sports car, Mullis had a sudden flash of inspiration. He swerved to the side of the road, grabbed

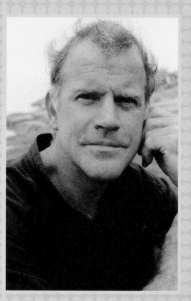

Kary Mullis

paper and a pencil, and furiously scribbled page after page of calculations. After a few minutes, he realized his idea really would work. He had come up with polymerase chain reaction—a way to clone billions of copies of DNA fragments quickly and inexpensively. This discovery was critical to DNA fingerprinting and to labs doing genetic research. Mullis went on to win the Nobel Prize in Chemistry in 1993.

Alec Jeffreys was quiet and modest about his success, while Kary Mullis basked in the publicity that came with his discovery. These two scientists with very different personalities both helped accelerate the genomic revolution, each in his own distinctive way.

The year before Alec Jeffreys developed DNA fingerprinting, a U.S. scientist named Kary Mullis made his own groundbreaking discovery. Mullis developed polymerase chain reaction (PCR)—a fast, simple, inexpensive method for copying DNA in large quantities. Mullis's discovery was powerfully important for DNA fingerprinting. DNA evidence is often hard to come by. It may be as slight as a trace of saliva on a cigarette butt or a speck of dried blood on a knife. PCR can create a billion identical copies of a single piece of DNA in a matter of hours. This gives police lab technicians plenty of evidence to work with. But Mullis's technique has revolutionized more than DNA fingerprinting. PCR is used to clone DNA in virtually every laboratory that does genetic research.

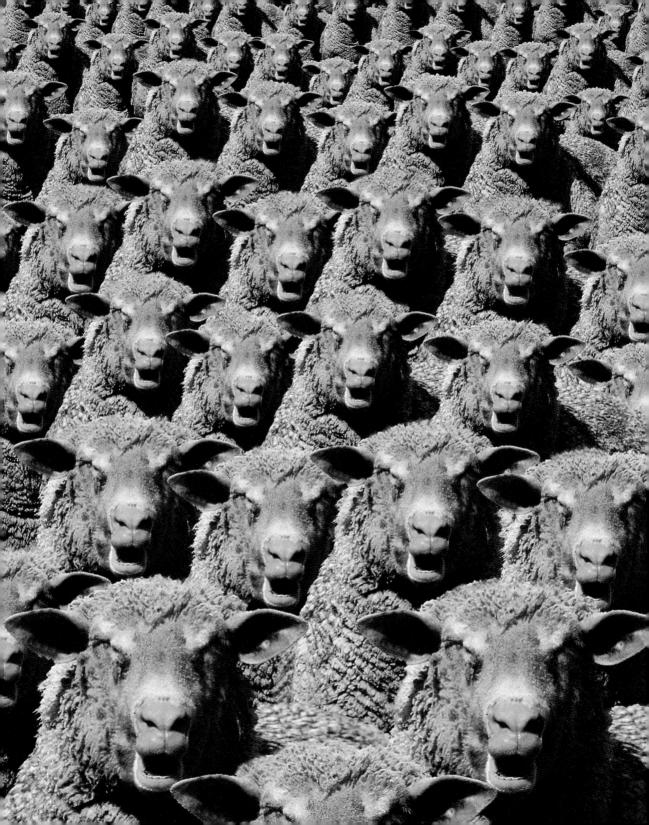

Chapter Nine

ENGINEERING NATURE

The genomic revolution involves animals and plants as well as human beings. Scientists are genetically engineering plants and animals to benefit humankind. One potential benefit is the cure and prevention of diseases.

Imagine eating a banana to protect yourself from a deadly disease. Before the genomic revolution, the idea of using the lowly banana to help prevent disease would have made people laugh. But it's a real possibility. Researchers are engineering bananas to produce vaccines that prevent infectious diseases such as tuberculosis and hepatitis B. Vaccines are weakened forms of disease viruses that build up a person's resistance to the disease. Instead of taking the vaccine in the usual way, through a needle, a person would just peel and eat a genetically engineered banana.

The deadly *Anopheles gambiae* mosquito is an even more unlikely tool to fight disease. These insects carry malaria, a disease that kills more than two million people each year. Most of the victims are African children under the age of five. Scientists have never been able to develop a malaria vaccine, but thanks to the genomic revolution, researchers may one day conquer this deadly disease another way.

A graphic artist's depiction of a cloned sheep (*facing page*) **illustrates the popular belief that clones are exact replicas. While cloned genotypes (genomes) are the same, phenotypes (physical expressions of genomes) can be different.**

In recent years, scientists have sequenced the genomes of both *Anopheles gambiae* and the single-celled parasite that causes malaria. When *Anopheles gambiae* bites humans, it transmits the malaria-causing parasite through its saliva. Scientists are trying to add new genes to mosquitoes' genomes that would keep the parasites out of the insects' saliva. If they are successful, their next goal will be to introduce these genetically engineered harmless *Anopheles gambiae* into the general mosquito population. Then the engineered mosquitoes could multiply, spread their altered genomes throughout the population, and eventually replace their malaria-carrying cousins.

These are just two of many health-related genetic engineering projects in the works. Others include corn engineered to produce cancer-fighting drugs and chickens engineered to lay eggs rich in disease-fighting drugs. As researchers sequence more plant and animal genomes, scientists will be searching for more ways to engineer them to benefit human health.

PRODUCING BETTER CROPS

Other scientists are focusing on engineering plants to produce crops that are more resistant to pests and more tolerant of extreme weather conditions. This kind of research started long before the Human Genome Project began. But the techniques developed by HGP scientists have helped agricultural researchers a great deal.

In April 2002, a year before the final draft of the human genome was published, research teams from China and Switzerland released genome maps of two widely grown varieties of rice. These maps are available to researchers free of charge on the Internet. By making this information public, the researchers hope to help scientists all over the world create new, more nutritious varieties of rice. This is important because one-third of the world's people rely on rice for half or more of their daily calories. This research should also help scientists studying wheat, corn, barley, and other grasses, since the genomes of all grasses are similar.

Genetically modified (GM) crops are especially important to the 800 million people worldwide who suffer from chronic hunger. Most of these people live in nations in Central and South America, the Caribbean, the Middle East, Asia, and Africa. As populations grow, poor nations must increase crop yields by growing more food per acre. In the past few decades, farmers have used improved fertilizers and pesticides to increase yields. But in some areas, these products have reached their limits. To grow more food for the world's increasing population, farmers must find new technologies.

GM crops offer hope. Indian chickpeas are a case in point. A large number of Indians are vegetarians, and chickpeas are one of their main sources of protein. But a tiny insect pest known as the pod borer has been consuming many of India's chickpeas before they can be harvested. These pests bore their way into chickpeas and eat them from the inside out. Sometimes they ruin a farmer's entire crop.

Who could stop these pests? Research scientists in India took up the challenge. When observing other plants, they noticed that the peanut was not vulnerable to the pod borers. The researchers altered the chickpea's genome by adding a gene from the peanut. The researchers hoped the peanut gene would stimulate chickpeas to produce a new chemical. If everything went according to plan, this chemical would prevent pod borers from digesting the chickpeas. After years of research, the scientists succeeded.

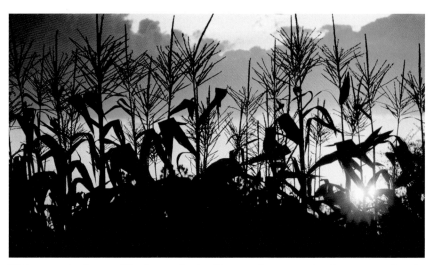

This genetically modified corn looks like regular corn. At the genetic level, however, it is different in a significant way. The genome of this corn has been altered to make it resistant to pests and disease.

THE DEBATE OVER GM CROPS

The genomes of other crops, such as potatoes, tomatoes, cotton, corn, soybeans, and rice, have also been engineered. Some of these GM crops have yielded more food per acre than ordinary crops. Others are more resistant to disease. Farmers can often grow GM crops more cheaply because the crops need less fertilizer and pesticide than regular crops. To many people, this sounds like a win-win situation—more abundant foods at lower cost.

But not everyone agrees. Some organizations in the United States and Europe object to GM foods. These organizations include environmental groups such as the Sierra Club, which has called for "a [halt] to the planting of all genetically engineered crops," and Greenpeace, which calls GM crops "genetic pollution."

According to opponents, the genomic revolution is moving too fast. It's transforming the world too quickly. People aren't thinking about the potential consequences, which could be serious.

Scientists use a kind of trial-and-error process when adding DNA to plant genomes. When they want to insert a new gene, they guess at a good location. If that position doesn't work, they try adding the gene in a different spot. They keep on experimenting until they find a position where the new gene works the way they want it to.

Even when researchers do locate the right position on the genome, they can't be certain that unintended side effects won't occur. What if these side effects turn out to be harmful or even deadly? Opponents worry that genetically engineered beans or apples or tomatoes could turn out to be "Frankenfoods" that damage people's health.

Once these GM plants are growing in fields, there is nothing to prevent them from pollinating normal, unmodified plants. Will the resulting offspring turn out to be "superweeds" that crowd out other plants? Opponents argue that new GM food products should be kept out of the fields and off supermarket shelves until scientists can assure the public that these foods are safe. Otherwise, opponents say, we risk upsetting the balance of nature.

According to supporters of GM foods, opponents' objections are based on fears, not facts. GM crops have been grown in more than forty countries on six continents for decades. In the United States, more than 90 million acres (40 million hectares) of GM crops are grown and consumed each year. Examples include Flavr Savr tomatoes, Roundup Ready soybeans, and Bt *(Bacillus thuringiensis)* corn. As a former FDA official points out, "There has not been a single mishap that resulted in injury to a single person or ecosystem" because of GM crops.

Objections are particularly strong in the nations that make up the European Union. Yet some European leaders have come out in favor of GM foods. Tony Blair, the British prime minister, condemns what he calls irrational protests against GM foods. "We cannot have vital work stifled simply because it's controversial," he says.

CLONING ANIMALS

Scientists perform genetic engineering experiments on animals as well as plants. They have been cloning animals since 1962, when John Gurdon, a biologist at Oxford University in England, used tadpole cells to create tadpole clones.

After Gurdon's groundbreaking experiment with amphibians, scientists' next goal was to clone a mammal. Over the next two decades, they made many attempts, mostly with mice. All of them failed, and eventually, most researchers gave up trying. They thought it was impossible.

Finally, Ian Wilmut and his colleagues at the Roslin Institute in Edinburgh, Scotland, proved other researchers wrong. In February 1996, a lamb named Dolly was cloned from the cell of a six-year-old ewe (a female sheep). These scientists inserted the nucleus from a ewe cell into a sheep egg cell from which they had removed the original nucleus. Then they stimulated the egg to make it divide and grow into an embryo, which they then implanted into the uterus of another, surrogate ewe.

Dolly died in 2003, after developing a lung infection. Most sheep live a few years longer, but many die of similar infections. One of the doctors who helped clone Dolly said that her death probably had nothing to do with the fact that she was a clone, but other scientists disagree.

The birth of Dolly began a parade of cloned mammals: a mouse in 1997, a cow the next year, a pig in 2000, a cat in 2001. Why clone animals? Money is one reason. Imagine a prize milk cow or a prize hog, the kind that wins state fair competitions and brings its proud owners a bundle of cash. Imagine scraping a few skin cells from these prize animals and using them to produce an unlimited number of clones, with each one as high quality as its "parent." Another reason to clone an animal is love. Imagine that a favorite pet has died. Imagine using the cloning process to replace that beloved pet with a clone.

The cloning process is still expensive and inefficient. Only about 2 percent of all cloned animal embryos result in live births, and many of those animals suffer from birth defects. But as scientists improve cloning techniques, success rates should climb and costs should fall.

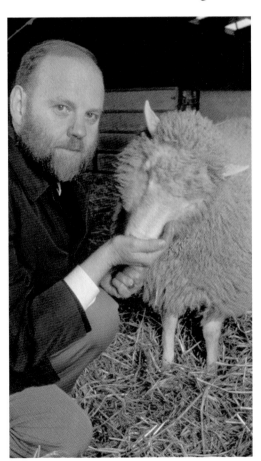

Genetic scientist Ian Wilmut feeds Dolly, the famous sheep that he cloned in 1996. She was the first mammal ever to be cloned from an adult mammal cell.

A COPIED CAT

As every pet owner knows, most pets have much shorter lives than people do. For instance, most dogs and cats live no longer than fifteen years. Because pet owners adore their animals, many are excited by the idea of bringing their loved ones back to life. That's why hundreds of pet owners have had samples of their pets' DNA stored for future cloning. PerPETuate, a company that offers this "gene banking" service, explains that "once animal cloning becomes a reality, you may be able to use the preserved DNA to clone your very special pet."

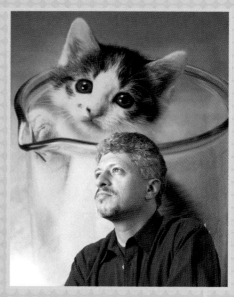

CC the cloned cat and Lou Hawthorne, head of GS&C, the company that funded the cloning

Another company, Genetic Savings & Clone (GS&C), sponsors animal cloning research. In December 2001, a GS&C-sponsored research team at Texas A&M University successfully cloned the first cat, which they named CC for "carbon copy." It took eighty-six failed attempts to finally bring CC into the world. Interestingly, CC does not have the same calico coat pattern as her mother. Cats' coat patterns are influenced by molecular changes while they are developing in their mother's—or surrogate mother's—womb.

Not everyone agrees that cloning pets is a good idea. Officials of the Humane Society, an organization dedicated to the compassionate treatment of animals, condemn the procedure. The Humane Society helps fund animal shelters across the country that care for unwanted animals and offer them for adoption. One of their officials said, "There are millions of cats in shelters and with rescue groups that need homes, and the last thing we need is a new production strategy for cats."

Bringing back extinct species is another reason to clone animals. In the science fiction movie *Jurassic Park,* a dinosaur is cloned from fossil remains. While this happened in the movie, it couldn't happen in real life. Scientists estimate that DNA survives for only about 10,000 years, and dinosaurs died out 65 million years ago. Even if scientists were miraculously able to find a dinosaur DNA sample, they would face enormous obstacles in actually trying to clone a living dinosaur.

But what about animals that became extinct more recently? A team of scientists at the Australian Museum in Sydney, Australia, have extracted DNA from an extinct animal, the Tasmanian tiger, that may be good enough to clone. The DNA comes from a pup preserved in alcohol since 1866. The last Tasmanian tiger on Earth died in a Hobart, Tasmania, zoo in 1936. When this animal died, so did the entire species. The preserved DNA has been damaged over the years and is missing certain sections of the genome. The Australian team is trying to fill in missing genes, create artificial chromosomes containing the DNA, grow live cells, and eventually re-create this vanished species, using a surrogate mother from another species.

Meanwhile, scientists are at work using cloning to save endangered species. In 1980 two banteng oxen fought with each other in San Diego Zoo's Wild Animal Park, near Escondido, California. One of the banteng, a male, died in the fight. Zoo officials froze skin cells from the dead banteng.

Twenty-three years later, on a farm in Sioux Center, Iowa, two banteng clones were produced from DNA from those skin cells. Scientists had transferred the banteng DNA into eggs from domestic cows, developed embryos from the eggs, and transferred them to the wombs of two ordinary cows that then gave birth to the clones.

The banteng were cloned because they belong to an endangered species. Banteng are nearly as rare as the giant panda. Fewer than five thousand banteng are left on the planet. Most live in Southeast Asia, where their habitat keeps shrinking as farmers clear forests to grow crops. People all over the world welcomed the news, but wildlife scientists urged caution. They noted that cloning is no substitute for protecting the habitats where endangered animals live.

CROSS-SPECIES CLONING

Imagine bulletproof vests made from spider silk produced by goats. Imagine human hearts produced by pigs. These projects and hundreds more like them are the specialty of cross-species cloning researchers.

In cross-species cloning, genes from one animal species are added to the cloned embryo of another species. The result is not a clone. It is a transgenic hybrid—an animal that appears ordinary but can do things that other members of its species cannot do.

For example, let's look at the goat that produces spider silk. It seems like an ordinary goat, and for the most part it is. The only difference is a few spider genes in its genome. The person who added those genes was Jeffrey Turner, a geneticist at a Canadian company called Nexia Biotechnologies. Turner added genes from a spider to the goat's genome and got the results he hoped for. The transgenic goat's milk contained the protein needed to make spider silk. Turner is developing a technique to extract the protein and spin it into thread.

Why create a goat with spider silk in its milk? The answer is strength. Ounce for ounce, spider silk is the strongest material on Earth. For that reason, it's in great demand for all sorts of products, from bulletproof vests to fishing line. Spider silk is impossible to get from spiders themselves in anything but tiny amounts, but Turner's goats produce it in generous quantities that are easy to harvest.

Turner's project does not involve human genes, but other cross-species cloning projects do. Some scientists are adding human genes to animal embryos to create medical products. To help fill the growing need for transplant organs, researchers are looking for ways to engineer pigs that can grow human tissue and, eventually, human livers, kidneys, and hearts. Researchers use pigs more than other animals because a pig's anatomy is similar to a human's and pigs can be genetically modified more easily than other animals.

By modifying pig genomes, researchers hope to overcome two major problems with xenotransplantation, or the transplanting of animal organs into humans: risk of organ rejection and risk of infection. The more like a human heart the pig's heart is, the less the chance that the human recipient's immune system will reject it. Infection is a potentially serious problem because animal cells can carry viruses that may end up being transferred to the human recipient.

CALLS FOR REGULATION

If the pig genome can be successfully modified to deal with rejection and infection, xenotransplantation will become a real medical possibility. But there will still be other problems to overcome. Some people object to using genetically engineered animals to produce human organs and other medical products. They say that putting animal organs into people is unnatural and immoral. Others say that it's cruel to raise animals simply to provide organs for humans.

Some people also object to researchers engineering animals to produce food products. They worry that researchers will somehow upset the balance of nature. As evidence, opponents point to a 2002 report from a National Academy of Sciences (NAS) panel that studied the biotechnology industry for the FDA.

The NAS report discusses some of the problems that might arise if biotech projects are allowed to get out of hand. For example, one biotech company wanted to market genetically engineered salmon raised on fish farms. The genes of these "supersalmon" were altered to make them grow faster and bigger than wild salmon. According to the report, if these "supersalmon" escaped from fish farms, they could easily overwhelm wild salmon, possibly even wipe them out. The report also mentioned dangers associated with transgenic milk, eggs, fish, and meat. Introducing them into the food supply might harm people by triggering allergies or other disorders.

The *New York Times* published an editorial reacting to the NAS report. It stated: "The most troubling problem identified by the panel is the creaking patchwork of laws and regulatory agencies that are expected to deal with a fast-moving technology. Congress needs to step in and clarify the authority and responsibility for regulating the products of biotechnology."

Both supporters and opponents of plant and animal genetic engineering agree that the federal government needs to regulate the biotech industry more closely. Researchers and scientists want minimal regulation that leaves them free to do their work. Environmental groups such as the Sierra Club and Greenpeace want stricter controls to make sure that the biotech industry's good intentions do not result in unintended harm. We can expect the debates over genetic engineering to continue as the genomic revolution moves ahead.

CONCLUSION

Where is the genomic revolution headed? Disturbing possibilities cloud the horizon. Before we review them, let's look at what we know for sure will happen. The genomic revolution will continue and scientists will keep sequencing the genomes of living species. Researchers will keep learning more about how human genes produce proteins and how those proteins develop into tissues, organs, and complete human beings.

Now for the probabilities—the things that stand a good chance of happening. Most experts agree that one day gene therapy will revolutionize the practice of medicine. They also agree that more varieties of GM foods will be produced and consumed, though not without protest.

This leaves us with the controversial possibilities. They include designing babies, enhancing people's genomes, using embryonic stem cells for research, cloning human beings, and discriminating against people on the basis of their genomes. These are the issues that generate the most heated debate. In the end, they leave us with tough moral and ethical dilemmas that may never be resolved.

Finally, there is one more certainty about the genomic revolution to think about. As it continues, we will continue to learn more about who we humans really are. Is this a good thing? Nineteenth-century Russian author Anton Chekhov thought so. He said, "Man will become better when you show him what he is like."

Scientists and researchers certainly agree. Every day they discover more about what people are like. But many scientists also say that we must keep a watchful eye on everything we do. As long as we carefully monitor this ongoing quest for knowledge about the secrets of life, we can realize the bright promises of the genomic revolution and hold the perils in check.

GLOSSARY

adult stem cell: a stem cell of an adult human being

allele: a specific variation of a gene. Different alleles result in differences in inherited traits such as eye color.

base pair: a pair of chemical bases (adenine and thymine or guanine and cytosine) that forms a rung of the DNA ladder

biotechnology: a branch of biology that uses genetic engineering techniques to alter the genetic material of living cells

cell: the basic unit of any living organism that carries on the biochemical processes of life

chromosome: a rodlike structure that contains DNA and is located in the nucleus of most cells. Humans have twenty-three pairs of chromosomes.

clone: an identical copy of an organism

designer baby: a baby produced through germline engineering, whose genes have been altered according to the parents' wishes

DNA (deoxyribonucleic acid): the molecule that contains genetic information and is passed from parent to child during reproduction. It is shaped like a spiraling ladder and is housed in the nucleus of most cells.

embryo: an animal in the early stages of development, from the time an egg cell is fertilized until it becomes a fetus with recognizable body structures

embryonic stem cell: a stem cell that originates from an embryo

enzyme: a protein molecule that makes chemical reactions occur more quickly or efficiently. One particular group of enzymes searches for and corrects mutations in DNA.

eugenics: a social movement dedicated to improving the human species by selective breeding

free radical: a highly reactive atom or group of atoms that can cause damage to DNA

gene: a sequence of base pairs located in a particular position in the genome that codes for the production of a specific protein or proteins

gene therapy: an experimental procedure to repair damaged genes or replace them with healthy genes

genetic discrimination: the act of judging, mistreating, or excluding people solely on the basis of the contents of their genomes

genetic disease: a disorder that is caused, at least in part, by mutations in one or more genes in the genome

genetic engineering: altering genetic material in the laboratory

genetic profile: a record of a patient's genome, used by doctors to predict disease and choose treatments to suit that particular patient

genetics: a branch of biology that deals with how living things inherit physical and behavioral characteristics through the genome and how these inherited characteristics vary from one individual to another

genome: all the genetic material in the chromosomes of an organism

genotyping: testing that shows the specific alleles inherited by an individual; often used to discover mutations that may contribute to a specific disease

germ cell: an egg or sperm cell

germline engineering: genetic engineering of egg or sperm cells (germ cells) or of a fertilized egg

Human Genome Project (HGP): the large-scale, international effort to sequence the entire human genome

in vitro fertilization (IVF): using laboratory techniques to fertilize egg cells and implanting the resulting embryos into a woman's uterus

"junk DNA": sequences of DNA in the genome that do not code for proteins. Despite its name, "junk DNA" has a variety of important jobs in regulating how genes function.

multigene disorder: a disease that is caused, at least in part, by several mutations in several different genes

mutant gene: a gene that has undergone a change in its nucleotide-base sequence

mutation: a random, accidental change in DNA's nucleotide bases. Mutations may be beneficial or harmful, but most have no effect.

nucleotide: one of the building blocks of DNA. A nucleotide consists of a sugar, a phosphate group, and a base.

nucleotide base: the portion of DNA that makes up the "rungs" of the spiraling ladder. The four bases are adenine (A), thymine (T), cytosine (C), and guanine (G). Genes are sequences of these bases.

oncogene: a gene that causes the body to generate new tissue to heal wounds and keep growing. Mutation of an oncogene may trigger cancer.

polymerase chain reaction (PCR): a method for quickly and inexpensively cloning fragments of DNA for research and for DNA fingerprinting

preimplantation genetic diagnosis (PGD): a technique used to check for genetic defects in embryos created by in vitro fertilization before implantation in a woman's uterus

protein: a large molecule created according to instructions from a gene. Proteins are the building blocks that make up cells, organs, and tissues.

replication: the process by which DNA copies itself so that, when a cell divides, each new cell gets an identical set of DNA

reproductive cloning: cloning for the purpose of creating human or animal life

sequencing: determining the order of base pairs in a DNA fragment, a gene, a chromosome, or an entire genome

single-gene disorder: a disease that is caused, at least in part, by the mutation of a single gene

single nucleotide polymorphism (SNP): a single nucleotide base difference in the genome sequence. Some SNPs (pronounced "snips") are responsible for physical differences between people, such as hair color, while others affect a person's chances of getting certain diseases.

somatic gene therapy: introducing new genes into the body's cells to cure or help control a genetic disease

stem cell: a generalized cell that has the ability to transform into different kinds of specialized cells, such as brain cells or blood cells

telomerase: the enzyme that maintains and rebuilds telomeres in stem cells

telomere: the tip of a chromosome. Each time a cell divides and the DNA is replicated, the telomeres become shorter. Because telomeres consist of "junk DNA" sequences, no vital gene information is lost during DNA replication.

therapeutic cloning: copying stem cells for use in gene therapy

transgenic hybrid: an organism that contains one or more genes from another species

tumor suppressor genes: genes that detect cancer cells and produce proteins to destroy them

vector: a device used to deliver new, healthy genes into cells as part of gene therapy. Most vectors are made from disabled viruses.

xenotransplantation: the process of transplanting the organs from one species into another

SOURCE NOTES

14. Susan Aldridge, *The Thread of Life: The Story of Genes and Genetic Engineering* (Cambridge, UK: Cambridge University Press, 1996), 23.

14. Robert Wright, "James Watson & Francis Crick," *Time.com*, March 29, 1999, <http://www.time.com/time/time100/scientist/profile/watsoncrick.html> (April 14, 2004).

14. J. D. Watson and F. H. C. Crick, "Molecular Structure of Nucleic Acids," *Nature*, April 25, 1953, <http://www.nature.com/nature/dna50/watsoncrick.pdf> (April 14, 2004).

25. Joannie Fischer, "21st Century Gold Rush," *ASEE Prism Online*, January 2001, <http://www.prism-magazine.org/jan01/gold_rush/gold_rush.cfm> (April 14, 2004).

37. Rex Chisholm, in discussion with the author, Chicago, Illinois, May 5, 2003.

42. Leon Jaroff, "Success Stories," *Time*, January 11, 1999, 73.

42. Sophie Petit-Zeman, "Gene Therapy Cures 'Bubble Boy,'" *New Scientist*, April 3, 2002, <http://www.newscientist.com/news/news.jsp?id=ns99992124> (March 8, 2004).

51. J. Travis, "Stem Cell Success." *Science News*, March 16, 2002, 163.

53. Chisholm, discussion.

53. Ibid.

62. Matt Ridley, *Genome: The Autobiography of a Species in 23 Chapters* (New York: HarperCollins, 1999), 243.

71. "Secrets of the Code," *CBSNEWS.com*, July 31, 2002, <http://www.cbsnews.com/stories/2002/09/24/6011/main523051.shtml> (March 10, 2004).

72. Rick J. Carlson, and Gary Stimeling, *The Terrible Gift: The Brave New World of Genetic Medicine* (New York: PublicAffairs, 2002), 265.

73. Ridley, *Genome*, 289.

73. Francis Fukuyama, *Our Posthuman Future: Consequences of the Biotechnology Revolution* (New York: Farrar, Straus and Giroux, 2002), 85.

74. Ibid., 72.

74. Richard Hayes, "In The Pipeline: Genetically Modified Humans?" *Multinational Monitor*, January/ February 2000, <http://www.ratical.org/co-globalize/mmGMhumans.html> (March 10, 2004).

77. Lee M. Silver, *Remaking Eden: Cloning and Beyond in a Brave New World* (New York: Avon Books, 1997), 236.

77. Silver, *Remaking Eden*, 236.

78. Kristen Philipkoski, "Why Cloning Didn't Happen in U.S.," *Wired News*, February 13, 2004, <http://www.wired.com/news/print/0,1294,62277,00.html> (March 10, 2004).

79. Gerald Ford, "Curing, Not Cloning," *Washington Post*, June 5, 2002, A23.

79. Silver, *Remaking Eden*, 98.

79. Michael Shermer, "I, Clone," *Scientific American,* March 10, 2003, <http://www.sciam .com/ article.cfm?articleID =00084EAF-2081-1E61- A98A809EC5880105 &sc =I100322> (March 10, 2004).

79. Silver, *Remaking Eden,* 98.

79. Ibid., 106.

80. President's Council on Bioethics, "Human Cloning and Human Dignity: An Ethical Inquiry," *Bioethics. gov,* July 2002, <http:// www.bioethics.gov/reports/cloning report/execsummary.html> (March 10, 2003).

80–81. "The Promise of Cloning," *Washington Post,* April 19, 2002, A24.

81. "President Bush Calls on Senate to Back Human Cloning Ban," *WhiteHouse.gov,* April 10, 2002, <http://www.whitehouse.gov/ news/releases/2002/04/200204 10-4.html> (March 10, 2004).

84. Kristen Philipkoski, "Negotiating Gene Science Ethics," *Wired News,* June 26, 2000, <http://www .wired.com/news/print/0,1294 ,36886,00.html> (March 11, 2004).

85. Richard Saltus, "Genetic Clairvoyance." *Boston Globe Magazine,* January 8, 1995, 14.

94. "Why Africans Are Starving," *Wall Street Journal,* September 17, 2002, A20.

95. Henry I. Miller, letter to the editor, *Wall Street Journal,* July 12, 2002.

96. Andy Coghlan, "'Irrational Protests' Harming Science, Says Blair," *New Scientist,* May 24, 2002, <http:// www.newscientist.com/news/ print.jsp?id=ns99992323> (March 12, 2004).

98. "The perPETuate Concept," *perPETuate, Inc.,* September 4, 2002, <http://www.perpetuate .net> (March 12, 2004).

98. Kristen Hays, "Genetic Copy of Cat Not a Copycat After All," *Chicago Sun-Times,* January 22, 2003, 32.

102. "Ranking Risks of Gene-Altered Animals," *New York Times,* September 4, 2002, A20.

103. "A Biological Understanding of Human Nature: A Talk with Steven Pinker," *Edge,* September 9, 2002, <http://www.edge.org/3rd_culture /pinker_blank/pinker_blank _print.html> (March 16, 2004).

SELECTED BIBLIOGRAPHY

Davies, Kevin. *Cracking the Code of Life: Inside the Race to Unlock Human DNA.* New York: Free Press, 2001.

Ridley, Matt. *Genome: The Autobiography of a Species in 23 Chapters.* New York: Harper-Collins, 1999.

Shreeve, James. *The Genome War: How Craig Venter Tried to Capture the Code of Life and Save the World.* New York: Alfred A. Knopf, 2004.

Silver, Lee M. *Remaking Eden: Cloning and Beyond in a Brave New World.* New York: Avon Books, 1997.

FURTHER READING AND WEBSITES

BOOKS

Cefrey, Holly. *Cloning and Genetic Engineering.* New York: Children's Press, 2002.

Fridell, Ron. *DNA Fingerprinting: The Ultimate Identity.* New York: Franklin Watts, 2001.

Marshall, Elizabeth L. *High-Tech Harvest: A Look at Genetically Engineered Foods.* New York: Franklin Watts, 1999.

Nardo, Don. *Cloning.* San Diego: Lucent Books, 2002.

Stock, Gregory. *Redesigning Humans: Our Inevitable Genetic Future.* New York: Houghton Mifflin, 2002.

WEBSITES

DNA from the Beginning
<www.dnaftb.org/dnaftb>
  This site presents the history of knowledge about the genome and brief, simple explanations of basic genetics concepts.

Genetic News and Links
<www.bio.davidson.edu/people/kahales/geneticslinks.html>
  Check out this wide-ranging collection of the latest news articles on the genomic revolution, along with links to sites that discuss the history of genetics, the Human Genome Project, cloning, and related topics.

Human Genome Project Information
<www.ornl.gov/hgmis/project/about.html>
  This official U.S. government site houses extensive information on all aspects of the Human Genome Project.

Hypermedia Glossary of Genetic Terms
<www.weihenstephan.de/~schlind/genglos.html>
  This compact, easy-to-navigate site offers both basic definitions and in-depth details about terms associated with the genomic revolution.

Your Genes, Your Health
<www.yourgenesyourhealth.org>
  This multimedia site gives quick, easy-to-understand details about genetic disorders and their treatments.

INDEX

ABOUT THE AUTHOR

Ron Fridell has written for radio, television, and newspaper. He also has written books about the Human Genome Project and the use of DNA to solve crimes. In addition to writing books, Fridell regularly visits libraries and schools to conduct workshops on nonfiction writing. He lives in Evanston, Illinois.

PHOTO ACKNOWLEDGMENTS

The images in this book are used with permission of: PhotoDisc Royalty Free by Getty Images, pp. 2–3, 94; © Jim Zuckerman/CORBIS, p. 6; courtesy of National Human Genome Research Institute, pp. 8 (right), 17; U.S. Department of Energy's Joint Genome Institute, Walnut Creek, CA, <http://www.jgi.doe.gov>, p. 8 (left); © Bettmann/CORBIS, p. 10; King's College London, p. 12; Bill Hauser, pp. 13; 15, 26, 41, 66; U.S. Department of Energy Human Genome Program, <http://www.ornl.gov.hgmis>, p. 16; © Getty Images, pp. 18, 50, 78; Gerald Baber, Virginia Tech/National Science Foundation, p. 20 (all); Bill Hauser/National Center for Biotechnology Information, pp. 23, 29; © Images.com/CORBIS, pp. 24, 34, 54, 70; Corbis Royalty Free Images, 29; © David Surowiecki/CORBIS SYGMA, p. 31; Mitch Doktycz, Life Sciences Division, Oak Ridge National Laboratory; U.S. Department of Energy Human Genome Program, <http://www.ornl.gov.hgmis>, p. 32; Jean-Marie Huron/AFP/Getty Images, p. 39; © Time Life Pictures/Getty Images, pp. 43, 86; © Peter Macdiarmid/Reuters/CORBIS, p. 46; © Kevin Unger/CORBIS SYGMA, p. 49; Robert Moyzis, University of California, Irvine, CA; U.S. Department of Energy Human Genome Program, <http://www.ornl.gov.hgmis>, p. 57; © Lester Lefkowitz/CORBIS, p. 60; Department of Energy Photo, p. 65; Advanced Cell Technology, Inc., Worcester, MA, p. 73; © Tim Bird/CORBIS, p. 82; © Reuters/CORBIS, p. 87; © Greg English/CORBIS SYGMA, p. 88; Sanford/Angliolo/CORBIS, p. 90; Najlah Feanny/CORBIS SABA, p. 97; © Kim Kulish/CORBIS, p. 98.

Cover: A. Pasieka/Photo Researchers, Inc.
Back cover: Robert Moyzis, University of California, Irvine, CA; U.S. Department of Energy Human Genome Program, <http://www.ornl.gov.hgmis>.

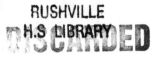